9/07

Your Complete Guide to

Total Hip Replacements

Before, During, and After Surgery

Jennifer Frantin, P.T.

An Idyll Arbor Personal Health Book

Idyll Arbor, Inc.

PO Box 720, Ravensdale, WA 98051 (425) 432-3231

Idyll Arbor, Inc. Editor: Thomas M. Blaschko

To the best of our knowledge, the information and recommendations of this book reflect currently accepted practice. The editors, author, and publisher disclaim responsibly for any adverse effects resulting directly or indirectly from the suggested medical practices, from any undetected errors, or from the reader's misunderstanding of the text. You must work with your doctors and therapists to make your hip replacement successful.

Library of Congress Cataloging-in-Publication Data

Frantin, Jennifer, 1965-
  Your complete guide to total hip replacements : before, during, and after surgery / Jennifer Frantin.
    p. cm. -- (An Idyll Arbor personal health book)
  Includes index.
  ISBN 1-882883-55-1 (pbk. : alk. paper)
  1. Total hip replacement--Popular works. 2. Total hip replacement--Patients--Rehabilitation--Popular works. I. Title. II. Series.
  RD549.F74 2004
  617.5'810592--dc22

2004009425

ISBN 1-882883-55-1

To the three most important men in my life:

Jim, Jonathan and Timmy

Acknowledgements

I would like to thank Dr. Stephen McIlveen, M.D. for his assistance in writing the chapter on the total hip replacement surgery. I would also like to thank my models and those who shared their total hip replacement success stories with me for use in this book.

Contents

Table of Figures

Forward

If you are reading this book, it means that you or someone you love has been suffering for some time. Whether from osteoarthritis, rheumatoid arthritis, avascular necrosis, or an old injury, when the bones that make up your hip joint fall into disrepair, pain can become a daily companion. The decision to undergo a total hip replacement can sometimes take years to make, but having a hip replacement can change your life. Unlike a person who needs a total hip replacement because of an accident or fall, you more than likely already suffer some degree of decreased or limited activity from the pain of your ailing hip joint. Of the over 600 total joint replacement patients I have worked with over the past fifteen years, I estimate 99% were thrilled with the outcome of their surgery and ready to kick themselves (figuratively, of course) for having waited so long to have the procedure.

Many questions surface whenever someone is faced with a major surgery, optional or otherwise. This book will attempt to answer these questions as well as give you useful and relevant information that will assist you not only with your decision to have the joint replacement, but also with your recovery afterwards. From choosing an orthopedic surgeon to the importance of exercise, this book covers all the major issues and topics you will face should you decide to have a total hip replacement.

Deciding to have surgery is a very personal and individual choice. Many factors play into the decision, including your age, general health, lifestyle, limitations from your hip pain, and your own individual personality. As with any surgery, risk is involved and there are no guarantees. Read the book and then discuss your personal situation with your physician to see if this surgery is right for you. I think you will find that taking the book along with you on your total hip replacement journey will help you tremendously in reaching your goal of being functional and pain free again.

Chapter 1

Introduction

Over the past fifteen years of working with total hip replacement patients, I have been continually stunned by the lack of information given to these patients both prior to the surgery and afterwards. Being a home care therapist, my patients have been seen not only by their own orthopedist, but also by at least one or two different sets of physical and occupational therapists before I arrive at their door. When I provide them with some of the information in this book, I am shocked by the number of patients who reply, "Wow, no one ever told me that!" So, if you are like me and believe that knowledge is a good thing, then this is the book for you.

Here is what is in the book:

Chapter 2 has stories about people who have had total hip replacements. Most people are somewhat doubtful about whether to have this surgery, thinking they can continue to "make do." I hope the examples of how much better off these people were after surgery will inspire you to

seriously consider the possibility that you might want to
have a total hip replacement.

After the stories I'll tell you about what happens when
you have a total hip replacement. Part 1 looks at preparing
for surgery. At the end of each chapter in Part 1 there is a
checklist you can use to make sure you have taken care of
everything you need to do before surgery. Part 2 looks at
what happens during and after your surgery. Of course, you
should read it through before your surgery so you will
understand what to expect. After surgery you can go back
and read it again to make sure your recovery is progressing
as it should. At the end of the book there are four
checklists: one for before your surgery, a second for your
hospital stay, and two more for you to keep track of your
recovery after surgery.

Use the pre-surgery checklist to mark when you have
completed the items in each chapter. Some of the checklists
are pretty easy to complete, but others may take some
effort. I suggest you do the work, because it really is
worthwhile to be as prepared as possible before your
surgery.

The checklist for the hospital stay will help you
remember all of the things you need to do during the time
you are in the hospital. It can be hectic, so this list should
help you remember everything.

The after surgery checklists will help you keep on track
during the first six weeks of your recovery. There will be
some discouraging times and the checklist will let you see
how much progress you have made.

Chapter 2

Stories from People
Who Have Been in Your Shoes

If you are on the fence about having the surgery and are looking for a little push to get you going, the following stories may help you find your way. These real life accounts of people who suffered from severe and limiting hip pain may be just what you need to help you make your decision to have surgery and have it now.

Arthur's Story
A Unique Birthday Present

Arthur left the hospital on his 70th birthday with a new hip and a desire to return to normal function as soon as possible. As a practicing psychiatrist, he was anxious to get back to his practice and his patients. He was adamant that a little surgery was not going to hold him back.

Arthur's hip pain began in 1959. He was hospitalized at that time. Aseptic necrosis was suspected but never confirmed. The pain eventually resolved itself, although not entirely, but Arthur admits to a high pain tolerance.

A few years before his total hip replacement surgery, Arthur's hip pain returned in earnest. The pain continued to increase over time and eventually led him to the decision to have a total hip replacement performed. When Arthur left the hospital on his birthday, he left walking with a walker. A mere two weeks later, he was using a cane. Arthur had two weeks of homecare physical therapy before continuing his rehabilitation with outpatient physical therapy. That therapy lasted only four weeks and he started walking without the cane during that time.

Arthur was also able to maintain his practice, returning to his office only three weeks after surgery. Although this was against the advice of his doctor, wife, and therapist, Arthur has proven that he is no worse for the wear. He did, however, agree to get up every half hour to walk and to do ankle pumps throughout his sessions.

Arthur readily admits that he has no regrets about the surgery. He enjoys a complete return to function, although he notes that he no longer jogs. But jogging aside, he is completely satisfied with his 70th birthday present, especially since he is now 74 and living life to the fullest.

Lucille's Story
From Pain to Piña Coladas

When Lucille's pain started to interfere with her life and her job as a bartender, she decided there was only one thing to do, have her hips replaced. Suffering from the wear and tear of years on her feet, both of Lucille's hips were extremely arthritic and caused her many sleepless nights and pain-filled days. Since her sister had already undergone the surgery for much the same reasons, Lucille decided to have both of her hips replaced, one at a time.

Before deciding on a surgeon, Lucille visited with many prominent orthopedists in her area. She was determined to find someone who felt right to her, someone who not only had a good reputation, but also was approachable, answered all her questions, and would be there for her from start to finish. Her efforts paid off and she found a surgeon with whom she was very happy. Her surgeon listened to Lucille when she announced that she did not want regional anesthesia, but instead wanted to be put out entirely with general anesthesia. He honored her request, not once, but both times she had her surgery.

Today, over two and a half years from her initial surgery, Lucille is feeling wonderful and is back to her life as a bartender. Although she is not limited in any of her activities of daily living, at 72 years of age, she still feels the need to be cautious. Her advice to anyone considering the surgery is three-fold: don't wait; research and choose the surgeon who is right for you; and follow the total hip replacement precautions and continue with your exercises every day. Excellent advice indeed!

Charlie's Story
An Easier Choice the Second Time Around

As a man whose jobs over the years were physically demanding, the wear and tear on Charlie's joints showed up at an early age. His hip pain started when he was in his 40s, but he just tried to ignore it and keep working. As his hip pain worsened, this became increasingly hard to do. With pain limiting his mobility and beginning to interfere with his job, Charlie decided to look into his options. A total hip replacement was suggested, but Charlie was not sure if he wanted to have a major operation. His doubts grew and he worried that the surgery might leave him worse off than his current condition, or even an invalid.

As time passed, Charlie found himself unable to lift even the lightest weights without excruciating pain. Time had run out for Charlie. It was impossible to ignore or work through the pain any longer. He opted for what he considered his last resort — he had a total hip replacement.

That was over twenty years ago, when Charlie was in his early 50s. He readily admits now that he is sorry he waited so long before having the surgery that changed his life. After his total hip replacement, Charlie's pain disappeared and he was able to resume the life that he had led before his hip problems had limited him so severely.

In 1998, when his other hip started to bother him, Charlie had no reservations about having a total hip replacement when it was suggested by his orthopedist. Determined to learn by his mistakes, Charlie scheduled the surgery right away and has never looked back. Now Charlie has two pain-free and functional hips. His first hip replacement has almost doubled its lifetime expectancy and Charlie is extremely satisfied with those results.

Donald's Story
The Total Hip Replacement "Poster Boy"

Donald prides himself as a man who can tolerate pain, but when the pain in his right knee got to be so bad that he was literally dragging the entire right side of his body, he decided to seek professional help. The x-ray of his right knee showed definite damage from arthritic changes, but nothing to match the severity of his pain, so his orthopedic surgeon suggested that they look at his right hip. Donald had been injured in the Vietnam War, requiring bone chips from his right hip to be used to fuse a section of his lower spine. When the x-rays returned, Donald's entire right hip appeared as a big blur on the film, with arthritis so severe that surgery was scheduled on the spot.

Being an avid weight lifter and golfer, Donald, who was 50 years old at the time of his surgery, was anxious to return to the sports he loved. Prior to surgery, he needed four Advil before the game, four at the nines, and four at the end of the game. His hope was to be able to give his liver a break and play medication free as soon as possible. Immediately following surgery, Donald noted that the pain in his groin, which radiated down to his knee, was completely gone. He did not even take pain medication while he was at the hospital. In nine weeks, Donald was back on the green, shooting a 92 in 18 holes without a single Advil. He also returned to weight lifting and continues to work out today without limitations.

Once the decision to have the surgery had been made, Donald's main concern was how much time he would have to take off from work. He owned his own dry cleaning business, providing the primary source of income for his family, so this weighed heavily on his mind. The day after his surgery, Donald was having a tough time believing that his leg, with this new titanium hip, would hold him up. But after one lap around the hospital wing with a walker, he graduated to crutches and left the hospital the next day. Donald returned to work on a restricted basis only two weeks after surgery.

Donald's life was enhanced so dramatically from this surgery that when his doctor asked him to speak at a seminar about total hip replacements, he jumped at the chance. Donald's advice to anyone considering the surgery is this: Don't wait to have the surgery. If you need it, do it. But he warns: Don't have the operation unless you are willing to put in the therapy time afterwards. Donald did very well with homecare physical therapy and then continued on his own afterwards. He still exercises every day and, as the fifth anniversary of his total hip replacement approaches, he is now getting ready to have his right knee replaced. He knows what's involved and he is ready for the challenge.

Ed's Story
Overcoming a Childhood Injury

In 1981, while riding his bike along a narrow road in the middle of Wisconsin's farm country, Ed was hit by a tractor and thrown into a drainage ditch. The sixteen year old's hip was badly dislocated and required hospitalization with four weeks of traction. The teenager endured many months of physical therapy following his release, but still experienced residual pain from the accident. For Ed, this was a life-changing event, but one that he learned to deal with and was determined not to let interfere with his life-long dream of becoming a priest.

Throughout his studies, Ed's hip problems continued to cause him mild discomfort. But he did not let this stop the pursuit of his dream. In 1990, Ed was ordained a Catholic priest. By the time Father Ed hit his 30th birthday, his hip pain had returned and, although he tried to ignore the pain and immobility, it continued to worsen. The heavy demands on his time helped him keep his mind off his own problems until his limp became so visible that parishioners became alarmed.

Finally unable to hide his disability, he decided to research his options. At first, his doctors told him that at 36, he was too young to have a total hip replacement. But as soon as an orthopedist saw the x-ray of his hip, which showed advanced arthritic changes stemming from his childhood injury, he assured Father Ed that a total hip replacement was indeed recommended.

Knowing that a total hip replacement was a necessity, Father Ed attempted to schedule the procedure, but a major factor that kept him from having the surgery immediately was time. Father Ed was responsible for not just one parish, but two, and his parishioner counted on him to be there for them. So, Father Ed put off the surgery for a few months, finally scheduling it when his hip pain increased so much that he could barely walk to the church.

Immediately thankful that he had undergone the surgery, Father Ed was surprised at how quickly he was able to resume some of his duties at his Church, including saying Mass. The pain he had lived with for much of his life was now gone. Father Ed is glad to be able to walk distances again, limp-free, and looks forward to a fulfilling life serving the Lord without further hip pain. He is now nearing his one-year anniversary and is feeling wonderful, with absolutely no limitations noted. His only regret is that he did not have the surgery sooner.

Father Ed's advice for anyone considering the surgery, no matter what age: Do It! Even if it means another surgery in 20 years, Father Ed is sure he made the right decision in opting for the total hip replacement now.

Harry's Story
From Eczema to Arthritis

Never in Harry's wildest dreams did he ever think that going to the doctor to treat one ailment would lead to another. Unfortunately, that is exactly what happened. When Harry's eczema was out of control, affecting his hands and feet so badly he found it hard to work or function, he sought the help of a dermatologist. Creams did little to help the painful rashes and fragile condition of the skin on his hands and feet. When his doctor started injecting him with cortisone once a month, the condition started to clear. Harry had no idea at the time that what was curing one problem was aggravating, if not causing, another.

A few months after the injections, Harry started to develop back pain. His job as a stagehand on Broadway kept him very active physically and the back pain was beginning to interfere with his work. When his chiropractor looked at his x-rays, he broke the stunning news to the physically fit 40-year-old — both of his hips were extremely arthritic. An orthopedic surgeon verified these findings, suggesting that the cortisone injections could have played a huge role in the deterioration of his hips.

Harry tolerated the pain for a few years, using pain medications to help him when needed. But the time finally came when the pain was too much to bear. On March 17, 1998, with the luck of the Irish on his side, Harry underwent his first of two total hip replacements.

Being young and healthy, as well as going to physical therapy for a month prior to surgery, helped Harry move rapidly to crutches only one day after surgery. His hip pain was completely gone, replaced with only surgical discomforts that would soon fade away. He continued his rehabilitation at home following his hospital stay and then spent several weeks in outpatient physical therapy to regain his strength and mobility. Returning to work, he found few limitations and decided to schedule his next surgery during Broadway's slow season in February.

Harry found he fared even better with his second surgery than the first since he was already familiar with the routine and was fortunate enough to have the same rehabilitation staff working with him. Again, he completed home care and outpatient physical therapy before returning to work. Now, three years following his second surgery, Harry notes that his only limitation is that he needs to hold onto something when he is getting up from a squatting or kneeling position. He has never regretted having the surgery, quite the contrary. His total hip replacements improved his quality of life tremendously and he would highly recommend having the surgery to anyone who is suffering from severe arthritis in their hips.

Harry is now four centimeters taller and about 20 pounds lighter than before his surgery. He no longer needs to rely on painkillers to get through the day and he is able to do whatever he wants physically. His favorite activity, playing with and chasing his young son, is now possible thanks to his two new hips and the skill of his surgeon.

Checklist for Deciding on Surgery

☐ These stories make it sound like surgery may be a good idea, so I'll keep reading.

Part 1

Preparing for Surgery

Chapter 3

Choosing your Doctor

Once you have decided that you want to explore the option of having your hip replaced, one of the first things you need to do is choose a surgeon. Although I realize that there are both female and male doctors, for the purpose of this book, I will use masculine pronouns when speaking of the doctor. To provide balance, I will use feminine pronouns when talking about therapists.

The choice of your doctor, or orthopedic surgeon to be more exact, is very important. Take your time, do the research, ask the questions in this book, and make sure you feel comfortable with your surgeon. His skill level and success rate is going to make a difference in the rest of your life.

There is a philosophy in this country which, although old-fashioned, still rings true for many: A doctor is god-like. With this way of thinking, it is unlikely that patients will want to "bother" the doctor with trivial things such as questions about their surgery or "waste his time" asking him to repeat what he just said because they did not understand one word of all that medical jargon. I admit, I fell victim to this mentality myself when I had my first child. I knew better, but I just did not want to sound stupid asking ridiculous questions or appearing to overstep my bounds by demanding certain treatment restrictions. Even when I finally got up enough courage to voice my request, I was lulled into silence again by the doctor's assurances that he knew what was best. He is after all, the professional, isn't he?

Doctors and surgeons are well-trained professionals who put in thousands of hours learning and fine-tuning their craft, but that does not automatically give them license to cut you out of the equation. The doctor you choose should treat you as an individual person, not just as "a hip." Just as you would expect a full explanation in language you can understand from a plumber before he started ripping away at your pipes, so too should you expect your doctor to answer any and all of your questions with his full attention. You are paying him to perform a service for you, just as you pay any other highly trained professional.

In the checklist at the end of the chapter you will find space for interviewing three doctors. You may not find the perfect doctor, so use the checklist to keep track of the good and bad points of each. It can be very hard to remember without having something written down. Filling this checklist out in pencil may be a good idea. Then, if you don't find an acceptable doctor in the first three tries, you can erase the worst one and go on to number four. You may not find the perfect doctor, but don't give up until you find one you really are comfortable with.

Checking References

When researching your doctor, talk with other people who have had him for a hip replacement. Ask them questions about your concerns: Did the doctor answer all your questions? Did you have any difficulty getting in touch with him if you had problems or concerns? Are you happy with the end result of the surgery? How was his follow-up care? Would you recommend him to a friend or family member? If you had to do it all over again, would you still choose the same surgeon?

Finding others who have already had the surgery is not as difficult as you might think. You can ask the doctor for a list of references or stop by an outpatient physical therapy office and inquire if they know of any of that doctor's patients who would be willing to talk with you. There may even be a joint replacement support group at your local hospital and much valuable information about different surgeons in your area and the surgery itself can be gained there. One word of advice — try to speak with people who are past the six-week point!

Checking Credentials

To check out the credentials of the doctor you are considering, you can call the State Board of Medical Examiners for your state or visit their website. The phone number is usually listed in the yellow pages just before the physicians' listings or under governmental agencies. To find their website, plug in State Board of Medical Examiners and your state into any search engine. Some states have slightly different names. The American Medical Association's list of contacts is available at this site:

http://www.ama-assn.org/ama/pub/category/2645.html

Your state board can provide you with important information on your surgeon's educational background and how long he has held his medical license in the state. Some states provide additional information. If your surgeon's license is new to a particular state and his education dates back many years, you might want to continue your investigation and find out why he moved. Even though a license has been suspended or revoked in one state, a person can still hold a license in a different state. While the state board may not be able to answer all of your questions, they are a reliable source of information on the quality of the service your doctor provides.

Meeting with the Doctor

The best way to know if your doctor is right for you is to interview him, so to speak, when you have your first appointment. Get the feel for the type of doctor he is. Does he rush in, speed around, and rush out, all before you can get out your first question, or does he give you time and listen? Does he use layman's terms when speaking with you or is he talking over your head? Does he appear to take what you say to heart or wave off your fears and apprehensions? Does he feel right to you? Just remember that, ultimately, you are hiring him; so if he does not do it for you, find the doctor who does.

Asking Specific Questions

First, let me say that the most important thing to remember from this section is to ALWAYS WRITE DOWN YOUR QUESTIONS BEFORE YOU GET INTO THE DOCTOR'S OFFICE. Why is this so important? Picture this: You arrive a few minutes early for your appointment. Your hip starts to bother you as you wait half an hour in the waiting room before they bring you back to an exam room. They ask you to undress, leaving a little paper thing behind for you to wrap yourself in. You finish and sit up on the exam table and wait...and wait...and wait. Finally, the doctor arrives and sweeps into the room with a comment about the beautiful weather we are having and then poof ... any and all questions you had are out of your head like magic. The doctor asks you how you are doing and all you can think to say is "fine."

This is not as unusual a scenario as you might think. In fact, it happens all the time. Your best defense is a complete and detailed list of all your questions. You can read the questions to the doctor right from the list. It shows you are a well-organized individual who is interested in his or her health and the doctor will probably respect that and treat you accordingly.

On your first visit, you might like to ask some general questions of the doctor such as:

1. What percentage of your practice is total hip replacement?

Gone are the days when one doctor did it all. Today, most surgeons specialize not only in one field, e.g. orthopedics, but more commonly, in one or two body parts. Many orthopedists may treat only the lower extremities (from the hips down) while others work primarily on backs and still others operate primarily on the shoulder, elbow, wrist, and hand. It is important to know the sub-specialty of the doctor you choose. This does not mean that a surgeon does not know how to do a total hip replacement if the majority of his practice is rotator cuff repairs on the shoulder, but if he only does five to ten a year, you might feel more comfortable with an orthopedist who specializes primarily in total hip replacements. It's also not a bad idea to ask how long the doctor has been in orthopedics and approximately how many total hip replacement surgeries he has performed during the past year and his entire career.

2. What percentage of your patients had a hip dislocation following the surgery?

This is a tricky question because the doctor does not have total control over his patients following surgery and therefore cannot be held responsible for every hip dislocation. Strict compliance with the total hip replacement precautions (which will be discussed further in Chapter 9) eliminates most of the problems with dislocation as long as the surgeon has done his part of the job correctly. A particularly high dislocation rate might indicate that the surgeon is a little off in his technique or that the appropriate follow-up care is not being provided.

3. **What percentage of your patients had a leg-length discrepancy following surgery?**

Often, this cannot be avoided. People need total hip replacements for a variety of reasons and some wait far longer than they should before they have the procedure done. When the surgeon removes the old bone to attach the new prosthesis, he has to estimate to the best of his ability, just where to cut to keep both legs as equal in length as possible.

If a person has been walking irregularly or limping for years, this sometimes creates a shift in the pelvis, which gives the appearance of two different leg lengths. Immediately after surgery and until you are walking again in a normal fashion, it is very difficult, short of an x-ray comparing the two, to tell if a leg-length discrepancy is true or caused by a pelvic shift. If, following surgery, you have a true leg-length discrepancy, it can be easily corrected with either an internal insert in your shoe or, if more pronounced, a lift secured to the bottom of your shoe. Any shoemaker can easily make the adjustments if needed. If, however, the discrepancy is caused by a shift in the pelvis, once you start walking with a normal gait pattern again, it should correct itself. It is for this reason that the doctor may ask you to wait several months before he assesses whether the leg-length difference is true or from a pelvic shift.

On the flip side of the coin, if you do have a true leg-length discrepancy before the surgery, the surgeon can generally correct it while performing the total hip replacement. Be sure to mention any leg-length concerns to your doctor.

4. What is the infection rate of your total hip replacement patients over the past five years?

Nosocomial infections (infections that are picked up in the hospital itself) are the most frequent complication of all hospital stays. Although your surgeon cannot be held completely responsible for such infections, a high rate of infection indicates a problem. Many things can contribute to increased infection rates from the simple, such as poor hand washing between patients, to the more complex, such as improper sterilization techniques. Good hospitals do everything they can to prevent the spread of infection and their efforts can be seen in the statistics on infection rate. If the infection rate of a particular hospital is high, ask the surgeon to perform the surgery at a different hospital where the rate is lower.

5. What is the revision rate of your total hip replacement patients over the past five years?

Revisions are needed in a small percentage of total hip replacement recipients. A revision is necessary if the hip surgery is not completely successful and something needs to be tweaked to make it right. Unlike infections, revision rates generally indicate the quality and skill of your surgeon. If a patient with a total hip replacement needs a revision within the first two years, there is a possibility the surgeon's technique was off somewhere along the line.

A revision may require the femoral head prosthesis to be replaced. This occurs primarily for one of two reasons. Either the prosthesis loosened within the femur or the angle of placement was off and, therefore, the ball did not ride smoothly in the socket. Extreme stresses on the joints following surgery can also contribute to the need for a revision but, if nothing extraordinary happened, an early revision indicates something went awry with the original surgery.

6.   Will I need both the ball (femoral head) and the socket (acetabulum) replaced?

The hip joint is a ball and socket joint, made up of the head of the femur (the large bone in your thigh) and the

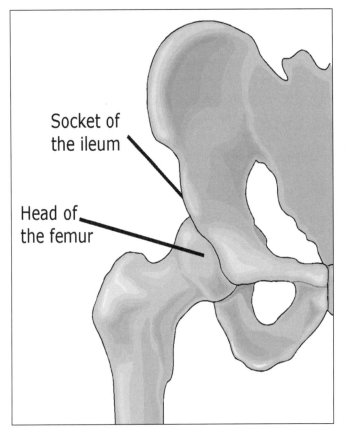

Socket of the ileum

Head of the femur

Figure 1: Illustration of the hip joint showing the ball and socket structure.

cup or acetabulum of the ileum (the large bone that primarily makes up your pelvis). (See Figure 1.) In some people, the head of the femur has been worn away from avascular necrosis or from the long-term effects of a previous injury, with no real damage to the acetabulum or socket.

In these cases, only the ball or femoral head is replaced, leaving the socket as is. In most cases, especially arthritis, both the ball and the socket have to be replaced. This does not really influence the rehabilitation or the recovery following surgery, but it is always wise to know just what you're getting!

7. **What is the current prosthesis made out of and what is the life expectancy for the prosthetic? (In other words, how long can I expect this thing to last?)**

Over the past decade, the material used for making the prosthesis for total hips and other total joints has changed so often that if I write down what they are using today, it will probably be different by the time you read this. These days metal, plastic, and ceramic replacement parts are all being used. Along with new materials, there are many different techniques of attaching the hip prosthetic: cement, cementless, etc. Each of these techniques changes the post-operative course, so it is important to ask the surgeon how the hip will be secured and what that will mean to your rehabilitation. For example, cementless replacements mean that you will not be able to put weight on your leg for several weeks, while using cement means that you can put weight on the leg right away. Some doctors prefer the cementless technique because the bone actually bonds with the prosthetic and can form a longer lasting replacement.

I think the most important issue is finding a doctor you can trust, but if you are interested in knowing about the latest materials and techniques, here are some web sites that have been good at presenting the most up-to-date information:
www.orthoglobe.com (select the patient forum)
www.joints.webmd.com
www.howost.com
www.ceramic-hip.com

If you want detailed information about many kinds of hip replacement systems try this location on the howost.com site (type both lines of the address into your browser with no spaces):
http://www.howost.com/medicalprofessional
/productoverview/hipimplants.php

Because of all of the advances with materials and tech-niques, it is virtually impossible for the doctor to give you an exact time frame for the life of the prosthesis. None of the new prostheses have been around long enough for a long-term study, but on average, total hip

replacements last between 12 and 17 years. The newer
models have the potential to last longer, however,
maybe even 20 years or more. Mind you, all of these
numbers are averages and there are no written
guarantees.

8.   What type of anesthesia do you think I will get?

There are two different ways for you to receive anesthesia, regional or general. Between your medical
doctor, your surgeon, and your own personal
preferences, your team will decide what is best for you.
Both have advantages and disadvantages so you need
to give this matter attention.

With general anesthesia, strong drugs are used to render your body unconscious and immobile. As with the
administration of any drug, this can be a dangerous and
complicated procedure. The anesthesiologist will
monitor all of your vital signs closely to ensure your
safety while under the influence of these drugs. Even
when you awake, the drugs can leave you feeling
drowsy for days. But when you wake up, the surgery is
over, you've got a new hip, and you don't remember a
thing.

On the other hand, regional anesthesia avoids many of
the risk factors associated with general anesthesia.
With a regional, also known as a spinal or epidural, the
anesthesiologist puts the drugs directly into your spine

through a catheter. Because the drugs do not need to circulate through your bloodstream, the "hangover" effect from general anesthesia mentioned above does not occur. Occasionally a regional anesthetic will leave you with a headache or backache, though.

The anesthesiologist will also give you medication to make you sleep through the procedure so you will be unaware of what is happening during surgery. A small number of people choose to be awake while using the regional anesthesia. Some, but not all, doctors will allow this if you are one of the people who is interested in being part of what is going on during surgery. Be sure to review all options with your team of doctors to get the one you are most comfortable with.

9. How many times will I see you following surgery?

The biggest complaint I hear from my patients is the lack of follow-up care provided by their surgeons. It seems to many of them that once the surgeon has done the hip replacement operation, he feels his job is over. But that is not the case and your doctor knows it. You paid him for the whole enchilada — before, during, and after. You will probably go to the surgeon once after two weeks or so for the removal of the stitches or staples and again at six weeks. Your doctor should continue to follow your progress over the next year with periodic visits. You need to know that your doctor is willing to call you back when you have questions or concerns and that he does not ignore you after the surgery has been completed. On that note, please remember to give him adequate time to return calls. It may take a few days before he gets back to you. If the matter is urgent, make sure you alert the staff of its importance when you are leaving your message.

Checklist for Finding a Doctor

Doctor's names:

1. _____
2. _____
3. _____

1	2	3	
☐	☐	☐	Patients of this doctor recommend him for his ability to communicate.
☐	☐	☐	Patients of this doctor recommend him for his skill as a surgeon.
☐	☐	☐	Patients of this doctor recommend him for his follow up care after the surgery.
☐	☐	☐	I've checked on this doctor's credentials and everything seems to be in order.
☐	☐	☐	I am able to communicate well with this doctor and get all of my questions and concerns answered.
☐	☐	☐	This doctor is a specialist in total hip replacements with adequate experience in the procedure he will be using.

		The doctor was willing to discuss his success and failure rates on the four issues shown below. (If he will not discuss these issues, it's probably time to find another doctor.)
—	—	Dislocation rate.
—	—	Leg-length discrepancy rate.
—	—	Infection rate.
—	—	Revision rate.
☐	☐	His plans for which part of the hip joint to replace made sense.
☐	☐	The prosthesis he is planning to use has an adequate life expectancy.
—	—	After discussing my preferences, he recommends general anesthesia (G) or regional anesthesia (R).
☐	☐	I am comfortable with his anesthesia choice.
☐	☐	This doctor will be available for follow up questions and treatment.

I've selected _____ as my doctor.

Chapter 4

Choosing Your Hospital

Choosing a doctor and choosing a hospital go together because most doctors do their surgery in just one or two hospitals. In making your decision, the doctor is probably the most important, but you should make sure that the hospital is also acceptable. Here are a few questions you may want to ask:

1. **How many total hip replacements are performed at this hospital each year?**

   As with doctors, there is an advantage to be at a hospital where they are familiar with total hip replacements. That way the whole staff at the hospital will be able to give you better care before and after the surgery.

   If you are in a rural area where there are not many hospitals to choose from, it might make sense to consider going to a major metropolitan center to have the surgery performed. It may seem simpler and easier to have the surgery done close to home. However, if something goes wrong because the hospital or doctor does not have sufficient experience, any corrections required will probably make you wish you had made a different decision. Skill and experience do matter for this surgery, so make sure you have it done in the right place.

2. Are the staff responsive to patient needs?

Ask to visit the areas where you will be during your stay at the hospital. See how the patients are being treated. The staff should respond quickly to calls and be pleasant and competent in everything they do.

3. Are the physical facilities clean and comfortable?

You are paying $1000 a day. You deserve a clean and comfortable place. Take a look during your visit at the physical layout of the hospital to be sure you will be as comfortable as possible.

4. What is the infection rate of the hospital for total hip replacement patients over the past five years?

Nosocomial infections (infections that are picked up in the hospital itself) are the largest complication of all hospital stays. Improper practices at the hospital are the most likely cause of a high rate of infection. Since a high rate of infection is an avoidable risk, you should choose a different hospital if the infection rate is high. A doctor who chooses to work at a hospital with a high infection rate might not be the best choice either.

5. What are your charging procedures?

Check with the hospital to see what is covered under their daily rate and when a day officially starts. In some facilities the day starts at midnight. If you stay past midnight, that day is already paid for, so you don't need to rush around when you are ready to leave. Other hospitals have a day start at 12:00 noon, in which case, you need to leave by noon or get charged for another day. Knowing when your hospital starts charging for the day will help you with your discharge planning.

6. What services are not included in the daily rate?

Some services in the hospital, believe it or not, are not included in your $1000+ per day charge. The phone and television may be such items. Check with your hospital to see if fees apply to such items and if they need to be paid in advance, daily, or if you can pay at the end of your stay.

7. If there are problems, whom do I contact?

When doctors shifted to specialization about 35 years ago, the American Hospital Association wanted to make sure that the voice of the patient was not lost. All hospitals are now required to have a patient advocate or ombudsman. Although the title may vary from institution to institution, all hospitals must provide this service for their patients. A patient advocate, who can be either a paid employee or a volunteer, will act as a liaison between the hospital staff and the patient should a problem arise. Familiarizing yourself with the system and how it works at the hospital in which you intend to have your surgery will help you not only if a problem should arise, but also give you peace of mind before you even put one foot through the hospital door.

The goal is to make sure you are comfortable that the hospital will provide you with a good environment for your surgery and recovery. If you have any questions about the quality of the hospital, you should ask to see a copy of the latest official survey. They are required to show this to anyone who asks. If there are numerous citations, it is time to look for another hospital and probably another doctor who does not continue to practice in an unacceptable environment.

Checklist for Deciding on a Hospital

☐	The hospital performs enough total hip replacement surgeries to give me good care.
☐	I am comfortable with the staff.
☐	I am comfortable with the facilities.
☐	The rate of infection is low.
☐	I understand the charging procedures and the services that are not included in the basic room rate.
☐	I know how to contact the patient advocate or ombudsman if there are any problems. The contact name is _____ and the phone number is _____.
☐	I have chosen to have the surgery done at _____.

Chapter 5

Planning Your Surgery

There are two important parts of planning your surgery that will be discussed in this chapter. The first is making sure that you and your doctor both have all the information you need to have a successful surgery. The second is scheduling the actual date of the surgery. Since you have some flexibility in when the surgery will be performed, you might as well schedule it for the best possible time.

Working with Your Doctor

Working with you doctor means that both of you know enough to be comfortable with the surgery. For the doctor, there are certain pieces of medical information that he needs so he can perform the surgery safely. It is his responsibility to gather that information. If he misses something important, though, be sure to tell him. He will be asking a lot of questions about your general health. Do your best to answer the questions accurately. If that means you need to get information from one or more of your other doctors, be sure to do that.

Discuss all of the medications you are taking, including vitamins and herbal supplements. Many people feel that "all-natural" products do not need to be reported. They do. Some of them have interactions with the medications you will be given that are as significant as the interactions with prescription medications. You also need to discuss any special diet that you are on. Some foods (grapefruit is one example) significantly reduce the effects of some medications. If there are any questions about your diet, be sure to mention them to your doctor. The goal is to ensure that whatever drugs you are given for infection control, anesthesia, or pain relief do not have harmful interactions with your current medications. Some medications may need to be stopped altogether before surgery, such as anti-coagulants. Make sure you write down everything you are taking and give the complete list to all of your doctors.

Make sure that all of your concerns about surgery and the follow-up are answered before the surgery. Hopefully, you have been able to select a doctor who is willing to answer your questions. Take the opportunity to ask.

Scheduling Surgery

When scheduling your surgery, there are many things to consider. Below are some issues to consider when you are deciding the best time to have your surgery. Keep in mind that there may never be a perfect time, but this will guide you in choosing the time that is best for you.

Have your surgery at the beginning of the week if possible.

Having surgery early in the week ensures that you will get the most out of the hospital services available to you, such as physical and occupational therapy. Although most hospitals have some rehabilitation staff on duty over the weekend, there is no guarantee you will be seen over the weekend. Avoid such problems by scheduling a Monday or Tuesday surgery.

If you are going into a rehabilitation facility after the surgery, this may be less of an issue. You may miss some rehab time at the hospital with Thursday or Friday surgery, but you should have more chances for weekday therapy sessions at the rehabilitation facility.

Make sure your surgeon will be around for follow-up.

Make sure that your surgeon is not going on vacation right after your surgery. You will want to have the surgeon nearby and available to you should you have any questions, concerns, or problems following surgery. A covering doctor is just not the same as having your own surgeon around.

Make sure support will be available.

You will need a lot of help for at least the first six weeks after surgery. If you are counting on help from friends and relatives, make sure you schedule your surgery for a time they will be available.

Pick the best time of year.

Choose the time of year that you have your surgery wisely. There may be less going on socially in January or February, but if you live in an area with a lot of snow or ice, you may wish to delay surgery until the weather is a bit less risky. (Living in warm climates does have its advantages sometimes.)

Have the surgery fit into your work schedule.

On average, most doctors will not let their patients return to work for at least the first six weeks. Many factors affect this decision, including your age, general health, and type of employment. Obviously if your job is very physical, it will take longer to return to work than someone who sits all day.

Regardless of your occupation, the total hip replacement precautions, which limit your movement to reduce the risk of dislocation, need to be followed for the first six weeks. So even if you have a desk job, returning to work sooner may be difficult.

Transportation may also be a factor in when you can return to work. Long car or bus commutes or busy subway stations may need to be avoided for a longer period of time. Make sure that, if you are still working, you schedule your surgery in a way that allows you to miss a considerable amount of work time.

Have dental work done before surgery.

Dental work increases the risk of infection in a newly replaced hip joint. Many doctors are recommending that if you need dental work done, you should have it done prior to surgery. Check with your doctor to see how much time he wants to have between when the dental work is done and your surgery.

Allow time to donate some blood for your surgery.

It is a common practice to donate some of your own blood before a surgery to reduce the risks of blood-borne infections. Two units of blood is the recommended amount. Since you can only donate one unit at a time, it may take a few weeks from when you donate the first unit until you have your surgery. Be sure to take that into account when you are scheduling your surgery.

Have the surgery fit into your personal schedule.

Confirm that there are no major events, like weddings or graduations, that you would like to attend in the first few weeks following surgery, especially if you plan on going to a rehabilitation hospital. You are unable to leave the facility or the hospital for a few hours and then return. If you leave, it will be for good, so plan accordingly. Most insurance providers also require you to be homebound to receive home care services. If you can make it out of your home to attend an event, then you will not be considered homebound and all home care services will be terminated.

Make sure that you will not need to go on any long car trips during the first month or so following surgery. When sitting in a car for prolonged periods following surgery, the muscles of your hip and leg stiffen, leaving you feeling uncomfortable and sore. If a long car ride becomes unexpectedly necessary after surgery, make sure you stop often and get out of the car to reduce the stiffness from prolonged sitting.

Schedule no major vacations for the first three months or so following surgery. Leave yourself at least a three-month window before you plan any serious traveling or vacations. Even though you will be back to relatively normal function long before that, your body might not be ready for the stresses and increased activity levels usually associated with vacations. As pleasant and enjoyable as they can be, there are a lot of stresses, both physical and mental, associated with vacationing and travel. Of course, you can go on vacation during this time, but if you want to get the most out of your trip, it is better to wait at least three months.

Check your insurance.

Depending on your insurance and your particular situation, you may choose to wait until the beginning of a new year if you have not satisfied your deductible and the year is close to an end. If you haven't fulfilled your deductible, waiting a few weeks may permit you to pay only one deductible for your surgery instead of two and help you pay less out of your pocket for your surgery and follow-up care.

When you are scheduling your surgery, there are some other questions pertaining to your life following surgery that will help you make your decision on when to have the surgery:

1. How long will I have to follow the total hip replacement precautions?

Most surgeons require their patients to follow total hip replacement precautions for at least six weeks. This is because it takes at least that long for the soft tissue surrounding the joint to heal and give the joint more stability. (This will be discussed in more detail in

Chapter 9.) More conservative doctors may extend that time frame to three months or longer. Every patient is different and therefore it is up to the surgeon to decide on time frames for the precautions. Whatever he decides, it is best to respect and abide by his decision.

2. When can I drive a car?

As badly as you want to get back to your normal life, driving a car is not likely to be part of it for the first six weeks, especially if you had your right hip done. Ask your doctor, but don't be surprised if the answer is not the one you were hoping for.

3. When can I play golf or tennis or ski again?

Again, as much as you are dying to get back out onto the green, it may take a little longer than the initial six weeks of rehabilitation before you are swinging again. Some sports, like golf and tennis, involve a good deal of rotation at the hips. For this reason, some surgeons suggest waiting several months before returning to tennis and even up to a full year before golfing. Skiing, on the other hand, may be highly discouraged by your surgeon. Because of the risk of falls, some total hip replacement recipients opt to hang up their skis for good, while others tone down their adventures on the slopes. I personally know a woman from Austria who had her hip replaced at a young age, mid-fifties, and refused to give up the sport she had learned at almost the same age as she had learned to walk. She has been skiing with her replaced hip for the past sixteen years without incident.

Your surgeon should be able to give you an idea of when and if return to your sport of choice is recommended. Much of his decision will depend on your age, general health, and proficiency at the desired sport or activity. Provide him with enough information to make his decision a well-informed one.

Although you should try to schedule your surgery to best fit your needs, do not postpone the surgery too long. There may never be a "perfect" time and sooner is better than later, so do not use scheduling as an excuse to delay surgery. In the long run, you will be glad you did not wait too long.

Checklist for Working with Your Doctor

☐	My doctor has taken a medical history that includes everything I think is relevant to my surgery.
☐	I have told my doctor about anything I think he may have missed.
☐	I have told my doctor about all of the medications, vitamins, and herbal supplements I take.
☐	I have told my doctor about any special diet I follow.
☐	I know as much as I want to know about the surgical process and the follow-up.

(another checklist is on the next page)

Checklist for Scheduling Surgery

☐	My surgery is on Monday or Tuesday. OR I am planning to go into a rehabilitation center so it doesn't matter.
☐	My surgeon will be around for follow-up.
☐	My support will be available.
☐	The weather will not be a problem.
☐	The date fits in my work schedule.
☐	I will make sure my dental work is done before surgery.
☐	I will allow time to donate blood for my surgery.
☐	The date fits in my personal schedule: no major events, no car trips, and no vacations during rehabilitation.
☐	This is the best time from an insurance point of view.
☐	I will need to follow total hip replacement precautions for ____ weeks. I can do that now.
☐	I will not be able to drive a car for ____ weeks. I can do that now.
☐	I will not be able to play my favorite sports for ____ weeks. I can wait that long so my hip will stop hurting.

My surgery is scheduled for
_____ (day of the week)
_____ (date).
Check in at the hospital is
_____ (time)
_____ (date).

Chapter 6

Your Insurance Company and You

Recently, there have been tremendous changes within the health care industry that directly affect those who wish to have optional surgery, such as total hip replacements. Only a decade ago the typical stay in the hospital for any joint replacement surgery was two weeks. Now patients are sent home in four days or less after major surgery (way too soon in my opinion). Rehabilitation center stays are shorter and, when the patient finally does get home, home care services are cut back as well.

When I first started doing home care in 1988, it was typical to see patients with hip replacements at least three times a week in their home (and this was after a two-week hospital stay, too). Today, that is not always the case. Therapy duration used to bring you through the critical first six weeks at the very least. Now, six weeks may be considered excessive. To be sure exactly what coverage you will be getting, you should go through the whole hip replacement scenario to find out what is and what isn't covered by your insurance company. Often this will mean that you may have to make some compromises about which doctor you choose and what care you ask for after surgery, but being prepared beforehand may also save you many financial problems.

You will probably not be able to find out everything in one call to your insurance company. For example, you will be calling to check on potential doctors before you meet them, but you will not know whether your doctor recommends a rehabilitation stay until you know who your doctor is. That's what the checklist is for: to help you remember all of the questions you need to ask, even ones that need to be asked at different times.

Let's start with the doctor. You should start by asking how many pre-surgery visits are covered. You may end up paying for visits to check out doctors if you don't like the first one you visit, but in the long run it may be worth it. Before you visit a doctor, check with the billing personnel in the doctor's office to find out whether the procedure is completely covered by your carrier. Some policies state that they will pay only the "reasonable and customary" fee for any given surgery. You should ask whether or not your surgeon's fee fits within these norms and, if not, if he will be satisfied with what the insurance company pays him. If not, you are responsible for the remainder of the bill. With a surgery of this magnitude, that could be a lot of money, so it is worth investigating.

Also remember to check to make sure your anesthesiologist is covered under your policy. You will get a separate bill for all anesthesia-related charges, above and beyond what your surgeon is charging for the surgery. Check with your insurance company to make sure that the anesthesiologist who will be working with you is covered under your policy. Otherwise, you may be in for a very expensive surprise.

Your hospital stay alone will cost thousands of dollars. Some policies dictate what type of room they will pay for, private rooms or semi-private rooms. In some case, you may have to pay an additional fee to have a certain type of room. Find out how many days in the hospital are covered in your policy and what happens if you need more time at the hospital. Also check if your insurance will cover a private duty nurse if needed.

If you plan to go to a rehabilitation center, call your insurance carrier and find out what they allow and ask to get your rehabilitation visits pre-approved. Find out how long your insurance company will cover your stay in a rehabilitation center should you decide to go. Likewise, check how long home care services will be provided. Some plans allow home care only for those who are homebound. This makes a lot of sense, until you hear their definition of homebound. For some insurance providers, if you can get out the front door and down a few steps, then you are not homebound. You will probably be able to do these simple things before you are really ready to venture out three times a week, getting into and then out of a car, just to have an hour or so of therapy.

Perhaps you live alone or do not have transportation. Perhaps you need to have your surgery during the winter months and it is too cold or icy to risk going out. Some insurance companies do not care if you live on the fourth floor and there is no elevator. They do not take such things into consideration. So, before you have your surgery, find out what the requirements are for you to receive home care. This will help you in your post-hospital decision making as well. By the way, it is largely up to the home care therapist to determine whether or not you are homebound, so if you have any concerns about going to outpatient before you are ready, be sure to discuss them with the home care therapist.

When it comes to physical therapy, make sure your policy covers physical therapy in the home, or home care, as well as outpatient physical therapy. Some policies have limits on the number of physical therapy visits or sessions. Clarification of those limits needs to be made — is it a set number of visits per year or per diagnosis? Does it include home care and outpatient physical therapy together or is it a set number of visits for each?

There is a chance that your insurance may help with some of the changes your home will require to make it safe for you after surgery. This includes anything you might need following surgery to assist you with your activities of daily living while you recover, including, but not limited to bathroom aids like elevated toilet seats and shower chairs, elevated chairs, hospital beds, and dressing aids. You can also ask about personal emergency monitoring systems.

After you go through the home safety chapter, you probably should go back to your insurance company and check.

Checking out just what is covered under your policy is very important before you embark on your journey. By either reading your policy, which can be very confusing and misleading, or speaking to a customer service representative, it is important that all of these questions be answered before your surgery. Making sure that you are covered for the services you need, including home care physical therapy and outpatient physical therapy, is critical and will help you in making your decision for surgery.

The one thing I have learned through years of dealing with insurance companies is that the squeaky wheel gets the grease. Keep after them. If they tell you that something you need and think you deserve under your policy is not possible, keep working your way up the chain of command until you get the results you want. Do not give up. Remember to always get the name, phone number (including extension number), and position of whomever you are speaking with. This will ensure that if a problem arises later on, you can provide the name and number of the individual who assisted you when you called. Also record the date and time of your calls just to be complete. Dealing with your insurance company or HMO can be a frustrating experience, but keep trucking. They have invested a lot of money into your new hip and they really do want you to be back on your feet as soon as possible. In the long run, it will cost them less if they make sure that all goes well following your surgery, including providing you with the therapy you need.

Medicare coverage is, believe it or not, more conducive to rehabilitation. You should still find out as much as you can about what is allowed and what they will cover before your surgery, as the rules for Medicare often change. One example is that Medicare may cover only one assistive devise per hospitalization, e.g., walker, cane, or crutches. More than likely, you will need more than one of these items, but Medicare may cover only one and you will be responsible for any others at your expense. (Be sure to check with the ambulance squad in your town or local Red Cross unit to see if they loan out walkers or canes before you buy one yourself.) Medicare will pay for a 3-in-1 commode for the bathroom, but no other bathroom devices. This commode can be used by the bedside, placed over the toilet as an elevated toilet seat, and used as a shower chair. But, not all bathrooms can accommodate such a unit and individual pieces of equipment may be needed, such as a portable raised toilet seat and shower chairs without the side armrests which can get in the way.

Medicare is also good about physical therapy, covering rehabilitation centers, home care, and outpatient services for as long as it is deemed medically necessary. Changes in the system of what they will and will not cover are inevitable. Please verify with Medicare what is covered to make sure you have the most up-to-date information available before your surgery.

Checklist for Insurance

☐ My insurance company has approved the surgery. OR I will be paying for the surgery without insurance.
☐ My share of the surgery bill will be _____.
☐ The anesthesiologist I will be using is covered by my insurance.
☐ My share of the bill for the anesthesiologist will be _____.
☐ My portion of the bill for my hospital stay will be _____.
☐ My share of expenses related to equipment I will get at the hospital will be _____.
☐ Insurance will cover _____ days at a rehabilitation center. I will need _____ days. My share of the cost will be _____.
☐ I will need some modifications to my home (as described in Chapter 8). The total cost will be about _____. My share of the cost will be _____.
☐ Insurance will cover _____ hours of home health care services for _____ days. I will actually need _____ days. My share of the total cost will be _____.

☐ Insurance will cover _____ sessions of home therapy. I will need _____ sessions. My share of the total cost will be _____.

☐ I will need _____ sessions of outpatient therapy. Insurance will pay for _____ sessions. My share of the cost will be. _____.

☐ My share of transportation costs for therapy will be _____.

☐ I will probably need the following assistive devices after my surgery: _____

_____.

My share of the cost will be _____.

☐ I have discussed the costs with my doctor and he agrees with the figures here.

☐ I talked to _____ at my insurance company _____ on _____ (date). The phone number was _____. (You can write other insurance company contacts below.)

☐ Other expenses not listed here are _____

_____

_____.

My total bill will be about _____ after my insurance has covered its share.

Chapter 7

After the Hospital

The next decision you need to make is what you will do when you leave the hospital. There are two possibilities. You can go into a rehabilitation center for a while or you can go directly home.

When I started as a physical therapist 15 years ago, my first job was in a hospital and I saw many people who had just had total hip replacements. The average hospital stay for a total hip replacement patient at that time was two weeks. Today, you are lucky if you get four days! With the onset of DRGs (diagnostic related groups) and HMOs (health maintenance organizations), hospital stays for joint replacement surgery have all but disappeared. As the "mini-hip" (see Chapter 10) becomes more mainstream, hospital stays are sure to be even shorter.

What I used to do at the hospital for my patients with total hip replacements is now done in a rehabilitation setting or at home. If you are unfortunate enough to have your surgery on a Thursday or Friday, you might see a physical therapist only once before you are discharged. (If you have any say in the scheduling of your surgery, early in the week is best so you can get the most from your hospital days.) Transferring to a rehabilitation inpatient center is one option following your surgery. Depending again on your general health and age, your doctor might recommend a short stay at a rehabilitation center.

Rehabilitation Centers

Rehabilitation centers are like hospitals, in that you stay overnight at them, but they concentrate more on rehabilitation. Typically, at a rehabilitation center you will have two sessions of physical therapy a day and at least one session of occupational therapy as well. More specific lessons can be learned at a rehabilitation center than in the hospital, such as using the stairs, getting into and out of a car, and more advanced exercises. Sometimes, if your endurance and strength are particularly low, your surgeon might highly recommend a rehabilitation center stay. This gives you the added physical and occupational therapy you may need before you go home. At the rehabilitation center you definitely get more physical and occupational therapy than you get at home with home care. Many people have benefited from a few extra days in a rehabilitation center before venturing home.

Take note, rehabilitation centers are not all the same. Some facilities specialize in more acute problems, like recovery from joint replacement surgeries and the patient population comes and goes quickly. Other facilities cater to those with more chronic health problems, but also provide rehabilitation services to people with more acute needs. These centers, which are more like nursing homes than rehabilitation hospitals, may not offer as much in the way of therapy as a more specialized rehabilitation center. Be sure to find out the main purpose of the facility you intend to use. Don't be fooled by the name. Actually go to the facility if you can or find out about it from someone that had his or her rehabilitation done there. Even if you think you will be coming directly home following surgery, go ahead and choose a facility just in case you change your mind.

Here are some questions you can ask to see if the facility matches what you are looking for:

1. **How long is the average stay?**

    Between you and your doctor, you need to figure out the appropriate length of stay in the rehabilitation facility. Make sure the facility you choose is appropriate for that length of stay.

2. **What percentage of the day is spent in therapy?**

    You are at the facility to get ready to go home. In general, the more time spent in therapy, the better. You should also make sure that you are comfortable that the therapists are flexible enough to allow for your level of endurance. Pushing you beyond your limits to meet a pre-planned schedule is not appropriate therapy.

3.   What services are included in the daily rate? What services will I have to pay for myself?

You need to know what services you will be receiving as part of the daily rate and what services have an extra charge. You are looking for the services you and your doctor feel you will need at a price you (with the help of your insurance company) can afford.

Going Directly Home

You may not want to spend time in a rehabilitation center. Home care, right from the hospital, is another option. It is highly likely that you will have home care following a stay at a rehabilitation center as well. Here is a look at what you can expect from home care whether you decide to go to a rehabilitation center first or decide to go home directly from the hospital.

Home care services consist of a nurse to monitor your progress on a medical level, a physical therapist, a home health aide if needed, and sometimes an occupational therapist as well. Unless you request a specific home health care agency, the discharge planner at the hospital will assign you to the agency associated with the hospital. Some home care agencies require a nurse to visit you in your home if you are receiving any home care services. It may be only a single visit or the nurse may make multiple visits, depending on your individual situation, but be sure to check what is covered for home care services in advance. Home care physical therapy is not the same as outpatient physical therapy. Some insurance policies limit the number of home care visits. You need to know what that limit means: Is it the number of visits allowed per year or per hospitalization? Are nursing visits included in that number? What happens after I hit my limit?

Home Care Nurse

The nurse will be in charge of monitoring your blood pressure and temperature. She will also watch your incision site for any signs of infection. Depending on your surgeon, it may even be the nurse who removes your stitches. (Staples are generally removed by the surgeon.) Organizing your medications and making sure that you are taking the proper doses at the right time of day is also one of the functions of the nurse. If a home health aide is needed, the nurse may be the one who determines that and makes the necessary arrangements. Nurses can also assist with starting a Meals On Wheels program for you (where hot food is delivered to your doorstep every day) or provide information on a home alert safety monitoring system (a necklace-like device worn by someone who will be alone most of the day to have instant and continual access to emergency personnel should an accident occur). Nurses are a wonderful source of information about what is available in your community to assist you while you are recovering.

Home Care Physical Therapist

The physical therapist will continue the program you began at the hospital or rehabilitation center, progressing you along as appropriate. She will work with you to make sure you can get around in your home. Some of the most difficult aspects will be getting in and out of bed, using the bathroom, and taking a shower. Your doctor will be able to suggest a therapist (or therapy service) to provide this care. Make sure the arrangements are in place before your surgery so that you will not have to worry about this during your recovery. You might want to talk to your therapist before you make a decision to be sure you and the therapist have compatible goals for your recovery.

Home Health Aides

Sometimes following a total hip replacement, a home health aide is placed in the home. Most insurance companies, including Medicare, limit the time allotted per patient to two hours, three times a week. More time may be available if it is needed desperately, but that would be determined by the nurse. You can also ask for additional hours and pay for them yourself.

Think about what you will need the aide to do for you. A lot depends on whether you have other people helping out with your care. Ask specific questions if you have any doubts about what an aide can and cannot do for you. All aides can help you with grooming, bathing, and dressing. Most will do cooking, limited cleaning, and washing clothes. Depending on the aide you get and the agency, some aides can even do light grocery shopping for you. Each agency is different, so it is important that you ask questions and find a service that fits your needs.

A lot of negative press has been circulating recently about the safety of home health aides. In many states, licensing of home health aides is now underway. This prevents people with questionable histories from taking jobs as home health aides. If you ever have any questions or concerns about the home health aides that come into your home, do not hesitate to call the agency that employs them. If you suspect anything is missing from your home, call the police immediately. It is extremely unfortunate to have to even think about such things, but it has happened. Better to be safe than sorry.

Outpatient Physical Therapy

Another thing to plan for before you go into the hospital is whether you want to have outpatient physical therapy. The answer is often yes. Outpatient physical therapy can be part of your home care during the six weeks it takes your hip joint to heal. It can continue beyond that time to help you rehabilitate your whole body if you have gotten out of shape because your hip was bothering you too much for you to pursue an exercise program. Many different outpatient facilities may be available in your area. Some are privately owned, while others are part of big, possibly nationwide, chains. Make sure to visit a few facilities before you make your final decision. Hospitals are also a good option for outpatient physical therapy. You may even find a familiar face or two if you go to the outpatient center at the same hospital where you had your surgery. Some hospitals even provide transportation to and from their facility for outpatient treatments.

Your surgeon may recommend a specific outpatient clinic, but he cannot force you to go anywhere. If your first choice is different from his, question him about why he is recommending that particular facility. Use that information, along with the information you accumulated on your own, while making your decision. Whatever type of outpatient center you choose, remember you have the right to feel comfortable and confident in your therapists. Ultimately, the choice is yours.

Deciding Where to Go after the Hospital

Much of the decision on where to go after the hospital rests on your general medical health and your living situation. For example, if you are living with a healthy spouse or other member of the family, it will be more reasonable to assume that someone will be there to help you get out of bed, put on your shoes and socks, etc., than if you are going home alone. The set up of your home is also a factor in deciding where to go after the hospital. If you live in a three-story apartment without an elevator, a rehabilitation center stay until you have mastered the stairs may be a more prudent option than returning home right away. If you are the type of person who will not do exercises on your own without prompting and encouragement, then perhaps a rehabilitation center should be considered before home care. Each person is different and there are many different and individual factors to weigh in making the decision about where to go after the hospital.

Discuss your options with your family and surgeon beforehand. If you think you would prefer to go home and your doctor wants you to go to a rehabilitation center, ask him politely why he thinks it is necessary and then tell him what you choose to do. He cannot force you to go anywhere against your will. He can only make a recommendation based on his knowledge and experience. Yours is the ultimate decision.

Other Issues Following Surgery

There are some other things that you need to be careful about after your surgery that aren't obvious when you think about the surgery itself. The first is that there is an increased possibility of blood clots forming in your leg. This is handled in two ways: exercise and medication. Your physical therapist will give you a set of exercises that will keep your leg muscles moving to move the blood back up your leg to your heart. In addition, your doctor may prescribe a blood-thinning medication, which also improves the chances of a successful recovery.

The second consideration involves visits to the dentist. You should take antibiotics any time you have dental work done, even routine cleaning. Infections in the mouth seem to get into the bloodstream more readily than infections in other places. Your new hip joint is vulnerable to infection, so you need to be as careful as possible regarding infections for the first year at least. Taking antibiotics when you go to the dentist seems to help.

Checklist for After Surgery

☐   I have decided to go directly home after surgery.
    OR
☐   I will be spending _____ days at the rehabilitation center: _____.
    (Fill out the checklist for the rehabilitation center on the next page.)

☐   I have found a nurse for home health care following surgery. Name of person or service: _____.
☐   I have found a physical therapist for home health care following surgery. Name of person or service: _____.
☐   I have found a home health aide for home health care following surgery. Name of person or service: _____.

☐   I will need to take the following precautions:
    _____
    _____.

☐   I will need to take the following medications:
    _____
    _____.

☐   I have included the costs of home health care in the insurance checklist.

Checklist for the Rehabilitation Center

☐	The rehabilitation center is appropriate for people who have had total hip replacements.
☐	The average stay is _____ days.
☐	I will be spending _____ hours a day in therapy. (The more, the better.)
☐	I have included the costs of the rehabilitation center in the insurance checklist.

Checklist for Outpatient Physical Therapy

☐	I chose _____ for my outpatient physical therapy.
	OR
☐	I decided not to check on outpatient physical therapy at this time.

Chapter 8

Preparing Your Home

While it's good to get home following surgery, you need to make sure your home is ready for you. Hidden obstacles can lurk anywhere. Smaller rooms and hallways make walking a bit more difficult than in the big open corridors at the hospital or rehabilitation center. Most bathrooms were not designed for use with a walker. With a little planning, and some temporary rearranging, your home can become safe in no time. Do it before your surgery and have everything ready for your return home.

You may need a few special items to make your home safer, as described below. Before you buy any of these items, check to see if you can borrow them from someone or from your local ambulance company or chapter of the Red Cross.

Clutter

Get rid of clutter. Sometimes, especially when you have been busy with other things like surgery, clutter magically appears. It is best to keep your main walking and living areas free from clutter. This helps to maintain a safe environment for all of the walking you will be doing around the house. The larger your area to walk, the better. Stairs are particularly a problem if cluttered. Have someone clear the stairs of all clutter before you attempt to climb them.

Pick Up All Throw Rugs

Too many people trip over loose throw rugs. When you have the additional feet of a walker, crutches, or cane to worry about, as well as your own feet, anything on the floor can be a hazard. Even larger area rugs demand caution when walking over or around them. Whenever there is a change in the surface of the floor, extra care must be taken to prevent falls. If you come home with a rolling walker, it is best to lift up the walker when you come to a new or uneven change of flooring. Be it from tile to carpet, hardwood to area rug, or even just a door jam, extra attention is necessary when walking over these obstacles.

Electrical Cords

Remove any electrical cords that run across the floor. Obviously, anything that runs across your floor, even if it is under a carpet, presents a safety hazard even when you are not just home from surgery. Extension cords and phone wires seem to be the biggest culprits since many older homes do not have as many outlets as state construction codes now require. Investing in additional outlets or running the extension cord around the exterior of the room is definitely preferable.

The Bathroom

More falls occur in the bathroom than anywhere else in the house. Small rugs in the bathroom should be used only when getting out of the shower and should have a rubber, non-skid backing. When not showering, these rugs should, if possible, be rolled up and tucked away. If you are living alone, this will not be possible, so use extreme caution and make sure the rug does not slip and slide or get caught in the walker.

Some bathroom doorways do not accommodate a walker in the regular forward position. If this is the case, you can turn the walker sideways with yourself still inside it and walk with slow, small steps sideways into the bathroom until you get through the doorway. Most bathrooms are small, so do your best to use your walker to get to the toilet and sink.

Do not leave your walker outside the bathroom and then grab onto anything and everything around you. This can lead to trouble. Most towel racks, for example, are simply glued to the wall and are not capable of supporting the weight of a person. If it goes down, so do you! In the smallest of bathrooms, you can probably still slide in sideways to get to the sink and toilet. Since there might not be enough room to spin around in there, make sure you are facing the right way before you start so your back faces the toilet.

Strategically placed grab bars are another way of assisting you in the bathroom. These bars can be used in the shower, near the toilet to help you get up, or on the walls if there is just no other way for you to get around in the bathroom. Make sure that grab bars are installed by a professional directly into the wall supports and not just glued on. They need to support your weight as you pull on them.

There are different ways to best utilize your bathroom safely, whatever its shape, so make sure your therapist helps you come up with a sensible way of doing so. Assistive devices such as an elevated toilet seat and modifications to the shower, as discussed below, will help make the bathroom safer.

The Toilet

If your toilet is low, you will need an elevated toilet seat. The total hip precautions require you to avoid bending your hip past 90 degrees. This even applies to the toilet. Your therapist will be able to help you select a toilet seat that is the appropriate height for you. You will also appreciate the added height because it is so much easier to stand up from a higher seat.

The Shower

You can't take a bath while following the total hip replacement precautions. Those precautions can make taking a shower a challenge, as well. A long-handled sponge helps you wash the lower half of your body without bending past 90 degrees at your hips or lifting your leg past that point. Other helpful devices are shower chairs, grab bars, and handheld shower head attachments. Your therapist can also help you select what style of shower chair would fit best in your bathroom and where to place grab bars if needed. Stall type showers are nice in that you do not need to lift your leg up high to get in, but they are sometimes cramped with a chair inside. This is when grab bars inside of the shower may help. Grab bars must be installed directly into the 2 x 4's that support the shower frame and not just glued to the tile. A professional plumber or handyman should be able to do this for you for a modest fee.

Glass sliding doors on tubs present a problem. The opening provided by the doors is sometimes not large enough for the person to fit through when using the shower chair. Temporarily removing the doors and putting up a shower curtain is a good idea. Once you are ready to step over the side of the tub again, the doors can be replaced.

Railings on Stairs

Make sure that the steps up to the house are in good condition and that there is a handrail on at least one side of the steps. Be it inside or out, stair railings are a must. Especially in the beginning, climbing stairs can be exhausting and frightening. Having a firm, supportive railing helps tremendously, both physically and psychologically. Since railings will most likely need to be installed by a professional, try to arrange their installation as much in advance as possible. You will be glad you did the first time you climb the stairs after surgery.

The Bedroom

If you need to climb stairs to get to your bedroom, you might want to look into renting a hospital bed for a few weeks or setting up a makeshift bedroom on the living level of your home. Not everyone will need to do this, but if you think you would rather not climb stairs for a while, it is easier to make arrangements before you go to the hospital.

Your Chair

Make sure you have a chair that is suitable for you to use upon your return. Because of the total hip replacement precautions, discussed in Chapter 9, you will not be able to bend at the waist past 90 degrees. For this reason, you will need a high, firm chair with armrests to help you get up without passing the 90-degree mark. In addition to the high chair, you will need a firm pillow or cushion to sit on. This additional height allows you a little more room to bring your center of gravity forward without bending at your hips past 90 degrees; thus making it easier to get up. You will need to bring this pillow with you to use in the car as well. If you are particularly tall, say 6' 2" or more, you may need to rent an elevated chair from a medical supply store. Call before your surgery to order it and make sure one will be available when you come home. Most chairs are rented on a monthly basis and your insurance company may pay for it. Be sure to ask.

Outdoor Walking

Whenever you walk outdoors, especially during the first few weeks following surgery, there are a few simple rules to keep in mind. First, try to walk only on paved or hard-packed surfaces. Stay away from grassy areas where holes and uneven surfaces can be hidden from view.

Second, watch out for Mother Nature's obstacles. Leaves can be particularly dangerous and slippery. Also watch for twigs or small stones that may throw off your balance. Try to stay inside during bad weather if possible. Wet surfaces can be almost as dangerous as icy ones.

Third, be aware of man-made obstacles. Most surfaces, even if they are relatively new, can have cracks in them. Make sure to be cautious about surface changes when walking on sidewalks, the street, or in a parking lot.

Finally, check the bottom tips of your assistive device when you return indoors. Make sure that no little pebbles have become lodged in the groves on the bottoms of the rubber tips on your cane, crutches, or walker. These small stones can make the foot of the cane or crutch slip on hard floor surfaces such as tile or hardwood. It is not a bad idea, as an added precaution, to occasionally pound the base of your cane or crutch hard against the floor to make sure the rubber tip is firmly attached.

Personal Emergency Monitoring Systems

Depending on your situation, you may benefit from the use of a monitoring system, such as Life Line, that provides you with the comfort of knowing you are not alone. With most systems, you wear a necklace or bracelet at all times. If you fall or find yourself in a dangerous situation, you hit the button on the device you are wearing and emergency service personnel are notified. There are many different service providers with different options, so check into what would best suit your needs. Most cost about a dollar a day. Some policies cover such services, while others do not. Even if your insurance does not cover it, this type of monitoring system can give peace of mind to those living alone or who are alone for a large portion of the day. If you are computer literate, you can find valuable information about the different companies offering such products by doing a search and entering the key words, personal emergency monitoring system.

Home Services

Check out the services provided by your community or local agencies. You might be eligible to receive hot meals from a Meals On Wheels program. You should also check with your house of worship to see if you can arrange home visits. If your mail and newspaper are delivered at the end of long driveway or down several flights of stairs, you might be able to arrange for these items to be delivered to your door for a short period of time.

Good, Supportive Shoes

In the home or in the hospital, it is imperative that you wear good shoes. Slip-on shoes or slippers present a major safety issue. While it may be easier to put on these types of footwear after a total hip replacement, it is extremely dangerous. Even wearing socks without shoes can be problematic as this can lead to falls from slipping on various types of surfaces, including tile, hardwoods, and linoleum. When buying shoes, look for lace up shoes with rubber, non-skid soles. Always wear shoes while walking and make sure the fit is snug. If your heel can slip in and out of the shoe, it is time for a new pair. Elastic laces also help keep your shoe snug while allowing you to slip then on and off easily. You may also find a long-handled shoehorn comes in handy when trying to put on your shoes while following the total hip replacement precautions.

For a few months following surgery, you may find that the foot on your operated side is swollen and may actually be a size or even two larger than the foot on your non-operated side. If this occurs, you may need to buy two of the same pairs of shoes in two different sizes to accommodate your swollen foot. Some of the high-end stores will actually sell you a pair of shoes with two different sizes, but it would serve you well to call before making the trip. Buying a second size of shoe is one of the things you can't do before surgery because you don't know what size you will need. However, you can contact the shoe store before surgery to plan buying the shoe if it is necessary. Eventually, your foot size will even out and you will be back to buying one pair of shoes at a time.

Checklist for My Home

☐	All of the clutter is picked up.
☐	All of the throw rugs are picked up.
☐	Electrical cords are out of the way so I won't trip on them.
☐	The bathroom is ready for me, including a safe shower and a safe toilet seat.
☐	All of the stairs, inside and out, have safe railings and are in good repair.
☐	I have a bed in a place I can get to easily.
☐	I have a chair I can use safely, one that is easy to get in and out of while still following the total hip replacement precautions.
☐	I've checked the places where I may need to walk outside to make sure they are as safe as possible.
☐	I have considered whether I need a personal emergency monitoring system. It will be there if I need it.
☐	I have arranged for as much as possible to simplify my life for the first six weeks after surgery including all of the home services I can get.
☐	I have safe shoes that I can put on and take off while still following the total hip replacement precautions.

Chapter 9

Total Hip Replacement Precautions

Because the integrity of your hip joint is completely disrupted during the total hip replacement surgery, precautions need to be followed to ensure the stability of the hip and prevent dislocation (the ball slipping out of the socket). In order to get to the diseased or broken femoral head, the surgeon has to cut through the joint capsule, the thick fibrous tissue that surrounds the joint. He also needs to get through some very big muscle groups. When the surgery is completed, the tissues are all sewn back together. However, it takes soft tissue such as the muscles and the joint capsule at least six weeks to heal. Until that time, these areas are vulnerable, and that is why the total hip replacement precautions are needed.

There are three basic precautions that must be strictly adhered to following surgery. Within each of these precautions are movements that should be avoided. Your physical therapist at the hospital will review these precautions with you, but knowing them beforehand is definitely beneficial. You really do need to follow them, without exception, for at least six weeks after surgery.

1.   Do not bend at the waist past 90 degrees.

This rule is easiest to break when you are sitting. When you are standing, it is very difficult to bend at the waist past 90 degrees without your hamstrings tightening first. Likewise, when you are lying in bed, unless you are totally propped up into a sitting position, your hips are not near the 90-degree mark. But when you are sitting, you are already at or near 90 degrees of flexion at the hip joint. For that reason, when you are following total hip replacement precautions, you need to sit on elevated chairs with pillows as shown in Figure 2.

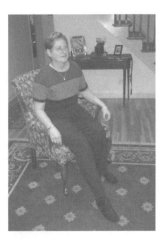

Figure 2: Sitting in an elevated chair to maintain proper flexion of the hip.

This decreases the angle at your hips and gives you a little more available movement while sitting. Otherwise, you would not be able to move at all without jeopardizing this 90-degree limit. When sitting, the knees should never be higher than the hips. Simply by straightening the operated leg out and bringing your knee down lower than your hip, you will decrease the degree of flexion at the hip on that side.

The extent of the elevation of the chair depends on your height and the type of chair. The best chairs to use are those that have armrests and are firm and high to start with. Adding a firm cushion or pillow to a chair like this may be all it takes. If you are particularly tall, say 6' 2" or taller, you might be better off renting an elevated chair from a medical supply store for the weeks you need it.

When you get up out of a chair, any chair, you need to lean forward to some degree to get your center of gravity over your feet so your body can rise up out of the chair. This is a problem for patients with total hip replacements because they are not allowed to bend at the hips past 90 degrees. The best way to get up from a chair or the bed while following these precautions is to stretch out your operated leg so that your knee is straight and your heel is resting on the floor as shown in Figure 3. This automatically decreases the degree of bend at your hip. The next step is to slide your bottom close to the edge of the chair and lean slightly forward

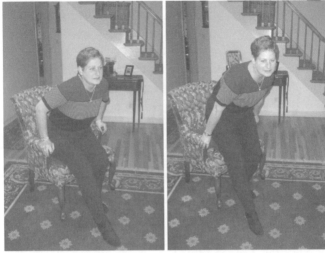

Figure 3: Getting out of a chair while keeping the hip at 90 degrees. Notice the pillow in the chair that was used to help keep the proper angle while sitting.

while pushing up with your hands on the armrest of your chair.

Here are some important things to remember. Be sure not to twist your body while getting up or pass the 90-degree mark at your hips. Avoid sitting on low or overly fluffy couches. Not only does this increase the chances of flexing or bending past 90 degrees at your hip when getting up, but since you will have an armrest on only one side of you, it will be harder to get up altogether. This can lead to twisting when rising, which is also not allowed. If you do find yourself in a situation where you are seated in a chair that is too low,

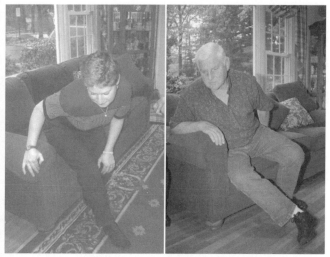

Figure 4: Examples of the WRONG way to get up. Get up without twisting if you can or ask for help.

don't panic. Scoot yourself to the edge of the chair, straighten out your knee to decrease the flexion at your hip and then lean forward while pushing up with your hands. Stop if you have any pain and use the assistance of another if needed. Just make sure that you do not twist in any way when rising. See Figure 4 for some examples of how not to get up.

Another part of the first total hip replacement precaution is that you may not bend forward or lift up your operated leg when you are sitting. Doing so would bring your hip past the 90-degree point. This means that if something drops on the floor, you cannot reach down and pick it up. An occupational therapist will show you how to use adaptive devices, such as a grabber, to help with this situation. It also means that you cannot bend over to put on your own shoe or sock or lift up your leg to do so. Be prepared to have some-one help you put on your shoes and socks for a while. Elastic shoe laces that do not need to be tied and untied every time you put on or take off your shoes are a necessary adaptation if you are living alone or have no one to assist you with this activity. They are available at your local medical supply store or on line from such sites as www.seniorshops.com, www.dynamic-living.com, or www.helpmates.com. A device to aid with putting on socks is also available, but it takes much patience and practice to master. If you do have someone to help you with your shoes and socks, take advantage of using them for the first six weeks at the very least. It is definitely the preferred way to go.

Another helpful and necessary piece of equipment is the elevated toilet seat. There are several different models, some that go over the seat like a commode and others that attach to the seat and are portable, so it would benefit you to think about what kind would work best for you. It works in much the same way as sitting in an elevated chair, by giving you a little extra room to lean forward to get up without passing the 90-degree mark. Most commodes and elevated toilet seats have adjustable legs so you can change the height to meet your individual needs. The elevated toilet chairs with arm rails give you the added advantage of being able to use your arm strength to help you get up.

Leaving the hospital or rehabilitation center may be your first time back in a car following surgery and you will need to bring a pillow to sit on to raise the seat height a bit. Taking a pillow along also helps when you are out because most public places do not have chairs that are high enough for you and a pillow may be just what you need to add the extra inches to make sitting safe. Further information about getting in and out of a car safely while maintaining the total hip precautions can be found in Chapter 17.

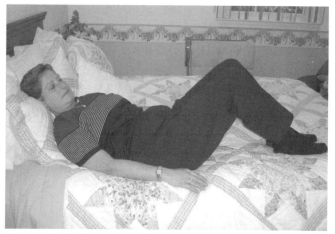

Figure 5: Lying down does not get the hips near 90 degrees, even with the knees bent.

Lying down, like standing, is not as much of a problem while following this precaution. When you are lying down, your hips are generally not at all near the 90-degree mark. Even when you bend your knees, you are not close to crossing the 90-degree mark as you can see in Figure 5. However, if you are sitting in bed with your back raised, you increase the angle at your hips and have to be careful not to exceed the 90-degree mark. See Figure 6. Don't make the mistake, however, of thinking that you don't need to worry about passing the 90-degree mark in bed. If you are sitting up in bed, it is basically the same as sitting in a chair, and the first precaution applies.

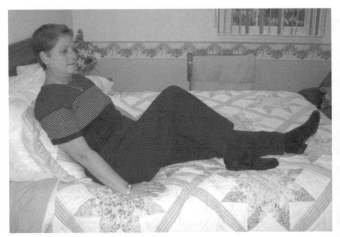

Figure 6: When you are sitting up in bed, you need to be careful about not bending your hip past 90 degrees.

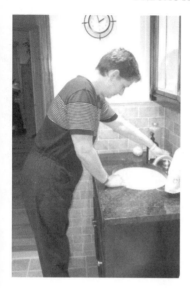

Figure 7: Standing at a sink does not cause much bending at the hips, as you can see in this picture.

While standing, it is fine to bend at the waist when, for example, you are brushing your teeth or washing your face. You do not have to stand rigidly, afraid of crossing that imaginary line, as you can see in Figure 7. As stated before, your hamstring muscles will more that likely stop you from bending before you come close to the 90-degree point. If, however, you are extremely flexible and can touch your toes, *don't do it*. You may not bend past 90 degrees no matter what position you are in.

Some doctors say 80 degrees is the maximum bend you are allowed. If your doctor tells you that, he means that you can bend at the hip even less than 90 degrees. The same rules still apply, but you need to be even more careful about getting out of chairs and cars.

2. Do not let your knees come together or cross the midline of your body.

Each knee has to stay on its own half of the body, as shown in Figure 8. This precaution becomes apparent to you the moment you wake up in the recovery room. A large, triangular pillow will be secured by Velcro between your legs. I affectionately call this pillow "the octopus" because it has eight straps to keep it snugly in place between your legs.

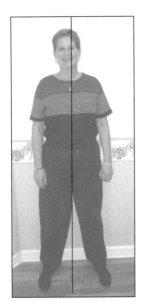

Figure 8: A line showing the midline of the body. The knee of the operated leg should never cross the midline.

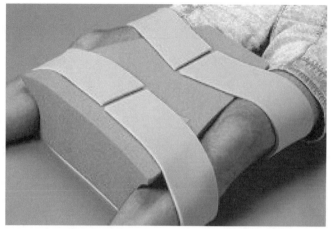

Figure 9: The legs are kept apart by the "octopus" whenever you are lying down.

Whenever you are lying down, especially to sleep, this abduction pillow must be between your legs (as shown in Figure 9) for the first few weeks following surgery. It is required to keep your legs from coming together, something you may have little control over when you are sleeping.

It is also a good idea to keep this pillow between your legs when you are sitting as well. Most people who have suffered hip pain over a prolonged period of time rarely cross their legs, but doing so now could dislocate the new hip, so the pillow acts as a physical reminder to keep the legs apart. You do not need to strap your legs into the pillow while sitting and can even turn the pillow sideways so it acts as a deterrent rather than as a brace.

As time passes, you may be able to replace "the octopus" with a regular pillow or, at the very least, pull the arms out of the octopus so you can get in and out of bed at night without the assistance of someone else. Be sure to check with your doctor before discontinuing the use of the abduction pillow.

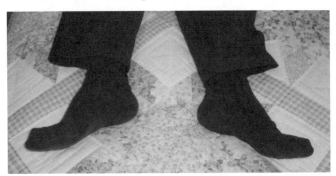

Figure 10: Feet pointed out. This is good.

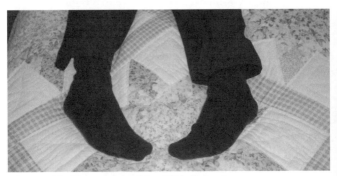

Figure 11: Feet pointed in. This is bad.

3. Do not let your leg rotate inward.

This is by far the hardest precaution for people to understand. When the surgeon does the surgery, his incisions through the muscles make the hip joint vulnerable to rotations after the surgery. This means that any rotation will push the ball of the new joint right up against the area of soft tissue (muscle and joint capsule) that is now weakened.

The key to this precaution is to keep your toes pointed forward or outward as shown in Figure 10. Do not let your toes roll inward as shown in Figure 11.

Although this is primarily important when lying or sitting, it is also important when standing and turning. Whenever you make a turn while standing, it is important to always move that leg first, e.g. if you want to make a right turn, move the right leg first. Keep this rule regardless of which leg is operated on. This ensures that your toes are always pointed outward. If you turn towards you operated side and move your unoperated leg first, steeping over or in front of your operated leg, you are rotating your operated leg inward, even though it looks as if your toes are still forward. The same is true in reverse. This precaution can be confusing, so have someone demonstrate this for you and it will all become clear. The pictures shown in Figure 12 may help, too.

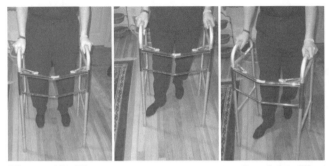

Figure 12: The proper way to turn to the right. First move the right foot toward the right as shown in the second picture. Then move the walker in the direction you want to go as shown in the third picture. Only when you are in this position can you move the left foot.

The risk of dislocation is minimal if you follow these precautions throughout the prescribed period of time, most likely at least six weeks. It is important to remember that there might be an occasion when you accidentally pass 90 degrees or violate one of the other precautions. If this happens, do not stay up all night worrying that your hip is going to pop out at any minute. If you do something that will dislocate your hip, you will know it then and there. Before you even get to the dislocation realm, you should feel pain. Listen to your body. Respect pain. Pain is, of course, very subjective, but you will know if you feel something that is sharp or breathtaking. If you experience pain, stop what you are doing. Analyze the situation. Are you bending at the waist past 90 degrees? Is your leg internally rotated or past the midline of your body? If it is and you can correct it, do so immediately.

If you have dislocated your hip, there will be no question in your mind. Get on the phone and call an ambulance immediately to take you to the hospital so your surgeon can pop the hip back into place. Most dislocations, and there are only a few of them percentage-wise, do not require further surgery. The surgeon is generally able to put the joint back into place in the emergency room, but the end result will be that you will now have to be in an uncomfortable and bulky abduction brace for at least six weeks. This entire scenario is something you really, really want to avoid, so try hard to comply with the precautions.

If you realize that you have not been following one of the precautions at some point but have had no ill effects, do not continue to ignore this precaution. Just because your body was able to tolerate the stress thus far does not mean that it will continue to do so. The very next time you do whatever it was you have been doing all along, it might just be the proverbial "straw that broke the camel's back."

Unfortunately, there is nothing you can do to speed up the healing of the soft tissue surrounding your hip joint. Many people are feeling so much better after a few weeks, better than perhaps they have in years, that they are tempted to do more than they should. Do not assume that because you are feeling strong and your hip is feeling fine, that it will be okay for you to "cheat" a little on the precautions. As good as you feel, your muscles and joint capsule are just not ready to take on the additional stresses that occur when you fail to follow these precautions. Do not tempt fate. You have come too far to spend the next six weeks in a brace because you dislocated your hip. Six long weeks, minimum!

As bothersome and annoying as these precautions may be, they serve a very real purpose. As anyone who has ever dislocated a hip will tell you, it's an experience you'd rather do without.

Checklist for
Total Hip Replacement Precautions

☐	I understand that I may not bend at the waist past 90 degrees and I have all of the things I need to follow this rule.
☐	I understand that I may not let my knees come together or cross the midline of my body.
☐	I understand that I may not let my leg rotate inward.
☐	Not only do I understand the precautions, I fully intend to follow them because I really, really don't want to spend one more second recovering from my operation than I need to.

Chapter 10

The Total Hip Replacement Surgery Itself

In a world where some people consider ignorance to be bliss, I must start off this chapter with a warning. Total hip replacement surgery is not a gentle, delicate operation. If you feel it would be better for you personally to not know what goes on in that operating room, skip ahead to the next chapter. If, however, you are from the school of "the more I know, the better," read on.

There are two types of total hip replacement surgeries being performed these days. I'll discuss the standard surgery first and then compare it to the newer "Mini-Hip" procedure.

Standard Hip Replacement Surgery

Because of the weight of your leg and the movements of your leg and hip during the operation, this surgery is a workout for all who participate. Before the surgeon can start, the anesthesiologist must do his part, administering whichever type of anesthesia has been decided upon by you and your doctor, including spinal or epidural technique, general anesthesia, or a combination of these methods. Prophylactic antibiotics are administered intravenously and a catheter is placed in your bladder for the purpose of monitoring urinary output during the surgery and the first few post-operative days.

Once you have been anesthetized, you are positioned by the surgeon and appropriate pads and cushions are used to hold you in a specific position for the surgical procedure itself. The entire leg, from the toes to the lower rib area, is then cleaned with various types of antiseptic solutions. Extreme care is placed on sterile technique in this "prepping and draping" part of the procedure.

Although there are several different surgical approaches for performing the actual operation, all are aimed at avoiding damage to the muscles and providing good exposure of the hip joint. The large hip muscles are typically cut and split with the least damage possible to expose the hip joint capsule, a thick fibrous structure that surrounds the hip and provides stability. Once the capsule has been cut, the upper part of the thigh bone (femur) can be dislocated from the hip joint.

The surgeon then uses a surgical saw to remove the top portion of the femur. If the hip socket, or acetabulum, also needs to be replaced, which is typically the case with people who have arthritis, the surgeon uses special instruments to prepare the area by removing a portion of

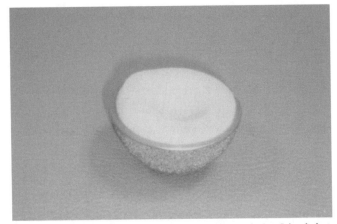

Figure 13: The acetabular component of the hip joint replacement.

the bone. He then inserts and attaches the prosthetic acetabulum component either with or without the use of bone cement (polmethylmethacrylate). A liner is then inserted into the inner lining of the acetabular cup as shown in Figure 13. The liner may be made of a very strong, high-density plastic or a ceramic material.

Preparation is then done surgically to the canal, or center section, of the upper part of the femur to allow for the insertion of the prosthetic hip. These implants, both acetabulum and femur, are either cemented into place or are inserted using a press fit method. The choice of which procedure to use depends on the age of the patient and, more importantly, the quality of the bone at the time of the surgery.

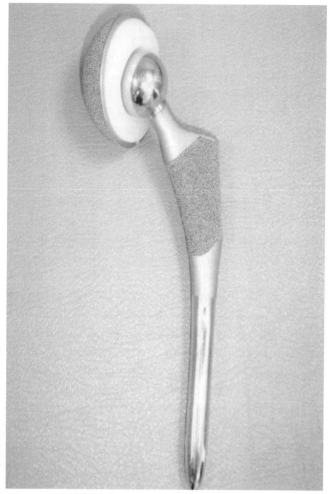

Figure 14: The femoral component of the hip joint replacement inserted in the socket.

The placement of the components in their proper orientation is extremely important in order to obtain good alignment, ensure appropriate leg length, and minimize the risk of dislocation. See Figure 14 for an example of what the femoral component of the hip joint looks like after it has been inserted into the socket. It has a long, narrow shaft with a thicker angular piece (neck) that connects to the ball area at the top of the prosthesis.

Once the prosthetic components have been inserted by the particular method chosen by the surgeon, the soft tissues that have previously been cut are now repaired using sutures. The skin incision site itself is either closed with surgical staples or a special skin sealing glue that has recently become popular. Immediately following surgery, you are brought to the recovery room to be monitored. A special device, known as an abduction pillow, is put between your legs to keep the operated leg in a stable position and prevent possible dislocation. When you awake and the recovery room staff feels it appropriate, you are transported back to your room to rest and wait for the first time standing on your new hip.

Although it sounds rough, and it is, the end result is a new hip with no arthritic changes to give you pain. The procedure itself takes several hours to complete, but in those few hours, your life will be reborn.

The "Mini-Hip" Surgery

There is a relatively new procedure being done by select orthopedic surgeons. This procedure is called the "mini-hip" or minimally invasive total hip replacement because the incision is much smaller than with the conventional total hip replacement. Instead of the standard surgery, which involves an incision of eight to twelve inches, the "mini hip" uses a different technique that allows surgeons to make a much smaller incision of three to six inches. Another technique uses two incisions (two inches and four inches). The hip prosthesis is the same as with conventional surgery, but the positioning and surgical techniques employed by the surgeon are different. A unique operating table and specialized training are needed before surgeons can perform this newer type of hip replacement.

Although less of the skin and musculature is cut during surgery, the total hip replacement precautions still need to be followed for the same length of time as with the traditional surgery. Soft tissue, such as the muscle and joint capsule, take time to heal, regardless of the length of the incision. Following the total hip replacement precautions prevents excessive stress on these tissues while healing occurs.

Surgeons who have performed the "mini-hip" have reported that in addition to the obvious cosmetic improvements, the benefits of the procedure include less post-surgical discomfort, less blood loss, shorter hospitalization, and a faster return to normal function. The extent of these claims is still unsubstantiated, but common sense will tell you that the less invasive a surgery, the quicker the recovery time. This procedure is still considered investigational by many, so be sure that you are comfortable trying something relatively new and that your insurance will cover it.

If you decide to find an orthopedic surgeon in your area who performs the "mini-hip," make sure you question him about his training in the procedure and ask how many of the procedures he has preformed, both with another, more skilled surgeon and on his own. Make sure your surgery is not his first solo attempt.

Although the "mini-hip" will probably be the surgical technique of choice in the future, it may still take many years before such surgery is commonplace. The new equipment and training that surgeons will need before advancing to the "mini-hip" procedure will prevent this from becoming an overnight substitute for traditional total hip replacement surgery, which has been proven successful for more than 40 years.

Checklist for Information about the Surgery

☐ I understand how my surgery will be done.

OR

☐ I have decided ignorance is bliss.

Part 2

Recovery

Part 2 of this book looks at the process of recovery after total hip replacement surgery. You should read it before your surgery to understand what you need to do for a successful surgery and recovery. The checklists for this part are found at the very end of the book. They are designed to help you keep track of your progress. Some days are discouraging, but seeing how far you have come will make the bad days much easier to handle.

Chapter 11

Your Hospital Stay

Nobody really likes to be in the hospital. We could all think of much better places to spend over $1000 a night. But the reality is, you need to go to the hospital to have this surgery. Don't worry, though, you're out of there pretty quickly. To make the most of the time you spend in the hospital, there are a few things you should know.

First, almost everything in that room (excluding the furniture and the TV), from the water pitcher to the egg crate under the sheets has been bought and paid for by you (or at the very least, your insurance company). Make sure you take all of it with you. Some of these pieces of equipment, like a urinal or bedpan may come in handy later on when you are at home. Be sure to take the abduction pillow, egg crate mattress cover, and anything else that they will likely dispose of once you have gone. They are yours, bought and paid for in full. Check with the nurse if you have any question about what you can and cannot take.

Speaking of nurses, not everyone in a white dress is a nurse these days. In fact, most nurses don't even wear white anymore. Many hospitals now provide surgical scrub outfits for the nurses and other hospital personnel, with differing colors for each department. Chances are, there may be only one or two nurses on your entire floor. Nursing is a field that was hit hard with the emergence of DRGs (Diagnostic Related Groupings) and HMOs (Health Maintenance Organizations). Because of these two influences, nurse's aides or assistants with significantly less training, who are paid only a fraction of the salary of an RN (registered nurse), are manning the floors. You probably will not know who is who by just looking, so you need to ask.

Make sure you know who the RN is on each shift and, if you have any problems or questions, ask one of the assistant nurses to get the real nurse for you. Chances are, you will not see the RN often because she is caught up in paperwork, but make it known that you want to see her and you will. Don't be afraid to ask for the credentials of the person giving you medications. This is your life and you are paying top dollar to stay in that hospital, so do not be deterred or be afraid about bothering someone. Just think of the service you would receive at a hotel where you paid $1000 a night! If you sneezed, they would be there with a tissue and a "God bless you" before you even realized it. In the hospital, however, you might have to wait hours for that same tissue. Even if it goes against your nature, be firm and vocal. Just because the hospital is trying to save money does not mean you should not be getting the service and attention that you have paid for and deserve.

As was stated earlier, the squeaky wheel gets the grease, so don't forget this during your hospital stay. If everything is not going as you would expect, tell someone in charge and don't stop pushing until things change to your satisfaction. Your patient advocate is another resource for making sure everything is done as it should be. Your stay is brief, but it doesn't need to be a bad memory. If you do have any problems with your hospital stay, make sure that when you get home and are feeling a little better, you write a letter to the president of the hospital outlining your complaints. The hospital is powerless to make changes if no one goes that extra mile and tells them what is really happening on the floors of their facility.

On the same note, if you had a great hospital experience, share that in writing as well. Patting the back of those who truly do a good job encourages them to continue to do so. Most hospitals strive hard to meet the needs of their patients. It is up to those patients to inform the hospital where they have got it right and where improvements should be made.

Chapter 12

The First Few Days after Surgery

The first day after any surgery is never a good one. More than likely you will be asking why you did this to yourself. Rest assured, it gets better. Each passing day brings more relief from the surgical discomfort you are feeling. In fact, the pain you had experienced over the past months or years is suddenly gone. To some people, the surgical discomfort is nothing compared to the agony they had been living with for so long.

By all means, however, take your pain medication! Don't try to tough it out or worry about becoming addicted. Your body just needs a little time to get over the trauma it has been through and, believe me, this surgery is a trauma to your body. If the pain mediation you are on is not agreeing with you (e.g., making you feel nauseous, lethargic, or just strange) tell the nurse or your doctor. There are many different pain medicines and everyone's body reacts differently. Do not relent on this point. Make sure you are heard and the situation is corrected immediately. There is no need for you to be any more uncomfortable than you already are. The nurse's job is to help make you feel better, not worse.

Very quickly, you will be back on your feet again. Your first steps will be with either a specially trained orthopedic nurse or a physical therapist. You may feel tentative about walking, but it is the best thing for you. Your doctor will have told you by then how much weight you are allowed to put on your operated leg and the therapist or nurse will guide and instruct you on walking with a walker or crutches. Do not be afraid to ask questions. If you are unsure about anything, speak up. More information on walking will be covered in the next chapter, "On Your Feet Again."

Depending on the type of anesthesia you had, you might feel a bit groggy for a few days. General anesthesia, in which they knock you out entirely, requires potent drugs that take some time to leave your system. Depending on your age, weight, and how long you were under, the effects of the medication may take as long as a week or more to disappear completely. Until that time, you may feel like you are in slow gear, but it will pass. If you chose regional anesthesia, you will experience almost no lasting effects from the anesthesia.

In the hospital, you will receive physical therapy and occupational therapy. The physical therapist will be teaching you how to walk using a walker or crutches. She will also be teaching you how to get in and out of bed and up and down from the chair. Total hip replacement precautions will be reviewed with you as well. A mild exercise program, such as the ones in Chapter 20, may be started, depending on how many times you get to have physical therapy. The main goal of physical therapy at the hospital level is to get you up and walking. Further therapy will take place either at home with a home care therapist or at a rehabilitation center.

Occupational therapy deals more with the adaptive equipment that will help you with your activities of daily living. Occupational therapists will show you how to use a grabber to get things off the ground, a device to help you get your socks on, and more. Since you need to use an elevated toilet seat, they will review your options with you and show you how to get in and out of a shower using a shower chair. Again, the amount that the occupational therapist can cover with you depends on the length of your stay and what part of the week you are in the hospital. Whatever training you do not get in the hospital will be covered either by the occupational therapist in the rehabilitation center or by the physical therapist with home care.

Chapter 13

On Your Feet Again

Following surgery, barring any complications, you should expect to be up on your feet that same day or by the next morning at the latest. A specially trained nurse or physical therapist will be with you when you take your first steps and will guide you in the use of your assistive device. Most likely, you will be using either a walker or crutches. Both of these assistive devices allow you to carry part of your body weight on your arms, reducing the stresses on your freshly operated leg.

Before your surgery, your doctor should tell you what amount of weight bearing he will permit you to use on your operated leg. This means that he will tell you, basically, how much weight you can put on that leg. There are four distinct weight-bearing categories: full weight bearing, partial weight bearing, toe-touch weight bearing, and non-weight bearing. Depending on the technique your surgeon uses, a total hip replacement patient could start off walking at any of these categories. Your doctor and your therapist will inform and instruct you on what you need to do for your particular surgery.

Full weight bearing status is now seen very frequently following total hip replacement surgery. This means that, from the start, you are able to put as much weight on your operated leg as you can tolerate, up to your full weight. You will still require the use of a walker or crutches for the first few weeks due to weakness of the hip musculature and as a safety precaution. Walkers come with wheels and without. At first, it may be best to start with a standard walker (without wheels), but after you start walking a bit better and more confidently, a wheeled walker may be a better alternative. Using a walker with wheels lends itself to a more natural gait pattern, for example walking one foot after the other in a continual pattern verses moving the walker and then taking one step with each foot. Again, it is a personal preference, but if you feel ready for a rolling walker after a week or so, be sure to ask your therapist or doctor about it. Likewise, if you do not feel comfortable changing to a walker with wheels, inform your therapist. Just one short note: Walkers with wheels also have brakes, so they only glide forward when lifted slightly. Once a person pushes down on the walker, the wheels lock and the walker stops. They are safe to use and do actually help with the return to a normal gait pattern.

At some point, usually after three weeks if you are in good general health, the surgeon may advance you to a cane. There are two types of canes, a straight cane and a quad cane. Although the quad cane has a wider base and gives more support, a straight cane is probably your better option. Unless you have pre-existing balance problems, a straight cane will suit your needs fully. The quad cane can be awkward due to its wide four-footed base getting into your way. Knowing your options is the best way for you to decide which cane will best suit your situation. You can also ask your therapist to help you try out both types of canes before you make your final decision.

The second weight bearing status is partial weight bearing. Generally partial weight bearing refers to less than full weight bearing. How much less is up to your doctor. He will probably give you a percentage to follow, such as 50% weight bearing. You would be surprised just how much weight is applied through your leg simply by putting your foot down on the floor. The best way to try to maintain the weight bearing percentage that your doctor has recommended is to take your body weight and multiply that by the percentage allotted. This will give you an amount, in pounds, that you are allowed to put on your leg. Get out your bathroom scale and experiment. You may be surprised how quickly that scale gets up there. The rest of your body weight must be taken up through your arms, as you press down onto your assistive device. If you are partial weight bearing, you will have to use a walker or crutches. You cannot move onto a cane until you have achieved full weight bearing status.

The third and most confusing weight bearing status is called toe-touch weight bearing. This term causes much confusion because people tend to think that as long as they only have their toes on the ground, they can put as much weight as they can tolerate through their operated leg. In reality, toe-touch weight bearing is closer to minimal weight bearing. What the term is supposed to indicate is that your toe or entire foot may rest on the ground primarily for balance purposes, but not to bear weight. It is very close to non-weight bearing, in which no weight at all is allowed on the operated leg, with the only exception being that the foot can actually touch the ground and does not need to be kept elevated. No doubt this confusion will continue until the wording is changed to a more accurate term, such as minimal weight bearing.

Finally, there is non-weight bearing. As mentioned above, this term indicates that no weight is allowed on the operated leg. As you can imagine, this is a difficult way to walk. You must use your upper body to hold your entire body weight with the walker or crutches while your unoperated leg swings through the air. Non-weight bearing status is often used for cementless replacement hips. As techniques change, it may be used for other types of surgeries as well.

Whatever your weight bearing status starts off as, your physical therapist will make sure you are walking according to the instructions. Additional weight bearing will be decided upon by the surgeon. In order to advance to a cane, you must first be full weight bearing and comfortable with the walker or crutches. When you do transition to a cane, do it in a slow progression. For example, start off using the cane only when someone is walking with you. Then when you are feeling more confident, use the cane for 20 or 30 percent of the day and the walker or crutches for the remainder. Slowly increase the amount of time you use the cane while decreasing the time with the walker. Eventually, you will walk only with the cane, but even then, keep the walker handy. Go back to the walker if you are particularly tired or sore and at night. No one is truly fully awake on those midnight journeys to the bathroom, so it is better to be safe than sorry.

Continue to use the walker when going outdoors for a while longer, as well, for safety reasons. When outdoors, try to stay off grassy areas, as there may be hidden holes and uneven areas beneath the grass. Whenever walking outdoors, watch out for Mother Nature's obstacles. Small stones, leaves, even cracks in the sidewalk are all potential hazards. Keep your eyes open. When you return indoors, check the bottom of your walker, crutches, or cane to ensure that no small stones have wedged into the ridges of the tips, causing a possible slipping hazard on tile and wood flooring.

Once you start to walk again following surgery, you will begin to feel better and better each day. Slowly increase the amount of walking you do daily. Before long, you will notice something incredible. You are walking and you don't have the pain that you had lived with for so long.

Chapter 14

Exercise and Recovery

Besides getting you up and about, your physical therapist will be teaching you different exercises to do on a daily basis. Exercise is extremely important following any surgery, especially orthopedic surgery. Immobility causes the greatest number of post-surgical problems. Muscle atrophy and bone weakening can start as quickly as the first day of immobility. Getting up as soon as possible following surgery helps to curb some of these potential problems.

A study on immobility was done several years ago using college students. After measuring their strength, the students stayed in bed for one week. They were allowed up only to use the bathroom and for one shower a day. At the end of this week, these healthy, 20 or so year old students lost 1/3 of their muscle strength. That's a lot of muscle for just one week. The study went on to watch the return of the student's strength and found that after one week of returning to normal activity with a light exercise program such as the one your therapist will give you, these students were able to regain half of what they had lost. Over the next week, they regained half of the remainder and by three weeks, they were back to their pre-study selves.

Realistically, you can therefore expect your recovery time to be at least three times as long as your immobility time. You are more than likely a few years older than those college students and perhaps have a few added medical problems, so don't be upset if it takes a little longer. The important thing to remember is that you can get back what you lost. Don't forget to factor into the equation your pre-operative activity level. Some people are barely able to move by the time they decide to have the surgery. This increases their rehabilitation time, but it is still doable!

Another important reason to exercise is to prevent blood clots. Blood clots form primarily in the veins of the legs post-surgically, which is why your doctor will probably put you into pressure stockings and may have you take a blood thinner for a while after surgery. When a blood clot breaks free into the blood stream, it will eventually end up in one of three places, none of which is good. If the blood clot ends up in your heart, it causes a heart attack; in your brain, a stroke; and in your lungs, a pulmonary embolism. As each of these conditions is immediately life threatening, prevention of blood clots is uppermost in the minds of the medical staff.

One simple ways to prevent blood clots is by getting up and moving around at least every hour. It is important not to sit during the day for longer than one hour without getting up and moving. Even if you just stand up and shift your weight a bit, it is better than sitting for a prolonged period of time.

Another useful preventative plan is to tap your feet as much as possible during the day. This simply involves tapping your feet as if to music 10 to 30 seconds, many times a day. With this simple tapping movement your muscles act as a pump to keep the blood flowing up towards your heart, which assists with the prevention of blood clots.

When blood leaves your heart, it travels to all the places in your body through very strong, muscle-lined vessels called arteries. These arteries get the blood where it needs to be without much effort, but after the blood has done its job, it needs to return to the heart through veins. Veins are flimsy, weak vessels that only have occasional valves to prevent the blood that's gone up (meaning towards your heart) from flowing backwards. Your veins rely on your muscles as they contract and relax to pump your blood back up to your heart.

If you are not walking as much as before or using your muscles through exercise, the blood from your feet and legs has a difficult time climbing up against gravity towards your heart. Picture a backpacker at the base of a mountain with his pack full of what he needs for his journey. If the mountain is too steep and the journey too difficult, he is going to have to give up some of the items in his pack to lighten his load. Just like the backpacker climbing a mountain, blood will dump off its non-essential elements (fluids) in the lowest, most gravity dependent area if it cannot get back to the heart. This is how swollen ankles develop. The danger lies not in the size of your feet and ankles, but in the thickness of the blood after it has let off this fluid. As you can imagine, the blood will be thicker once it has unloaded part of its fluid. This increases the chances of clotting. The good news is that the blood wants that fluid back, so at night, when your feet are level with your heart, the blood does its best to pick up this fluid and return your ankles to their regular state.

In combination with the toe tapping, alternating your position during the day helps to prevent clotting. You've heard the phrase, "too much of any one thing is no good." That is particularly true during rehabilitation of a total hip replacement. You need to alternate from sitting to standing, from having your feet down on the floor to up on an otto-man, from lying down to sitting up, etc. You can also move your feet back and forth when you are lying down or when they are elevated, like you are waving with your feet, as long as you don't let the toes turn inward. This does the same thing as tapping your feet and assists the blood on its way back to the heart.

Whenever exercising, try to remember that the phrase "no pain, no gain" may be true for an Olympic athlete, but does not hold true for you. You probably will experience some discomfort, especially in the area of the surgery where a lot of muscles were cut. What is important is to learn the difference between discomfort and pain. Discom-fort is dull and nagging while pain is sharp and sudden. Everyone's reaction to pain is different. Some people can tolerate large amounts of pain and some people are sensitive to the smallest twinge.

The point is to use pain as an indicator that what you are doing is harmful to your body. You need to avoid doing things that are damaging the recovery of your hip.

Listen to your body and stop if anything you are doing is painful. This is especially true for total hip replacement patients because of the dislocation factor. When you are exercising, if you have pain, stop. Try the exercise again later. You may have had a muscle spasm (or cramp) during the first attempt. It does your body and your muscles no good to work through a muscle spasm. If you still have pain during the second try, stop that exercise or activity. Check with your therapist the next time you see her. Perhaps you were in the wrong position for the exercise. No one works with you more directly and for a longer period of time than your therapist. She will be your greatest ally during your rehabilitation. Use her for whatever questions or concerns you may have. She may need to refer some of the questions to your surgeon, but she can answer most of them for you.

Endurance can also decline rapidly following surgery and immobility. It will be up to you to keep track of what you are capable of doing and increase your activity bit by bit on a daily basis. Your therapist will guide your activity in rehabilitation, but what you do on your own and how much more you do each day will really be up to you. What is desired is a nice, slow but steady progression of activity over the first six weeks. You are the only one who knows exactly what you do in one day. The best way to monitor and adjust your activity levels is to mentally record what you do one day and see how you feel the following morning.

Your body will let you overdo. I could probably go out and run a mile today but, chances are, I would not be walking too well tomorrow. You need to read your body and adjust your activities accordingly. Monitor what you do each day. If you wake the next morning with very little or no increased muscle soreness, then you can increase your activity level a bit. If, however, you awake with much increased soreness, it probably means you overdid it the day before and that you should cut back slightly on your activity. This does not mean that you should stay in bed or not do anything that day. If you do, then you will lose some of what you gained and, when you resume your activity, the chances are you will again be sore the following day. Can you see a bad cycle starting here? It is best to keep moving even if you are sore, just do a little less than the day before.

A lot of people experience increased soreness after their first trip to the doctor. Even if you do not think you are doing much while sitting around waiting for the doctor, sometimes it just takes a lot out of your body. Do not be surprised if this happens to you. Chances are you were not planning to go out two days in a row, so already your activity will be decreased. Just keep moving.

When you start your rehabilitation program, you will find that most exercises are done in groups of ten. You may be doing two or three sets of ten. This is different from one set of 30. The reason the exercise is divided up into sets of ten is to let fresh oxygen from your bloodstream get into your muscles between sets. When you do not relax the muscles enough to let the fresh oxygen in, your muscles need to rely on the stored up energy within them. Doing this requires a chemical reaction to take place in the muscle fibers, which produces lactic acid. It is lactic acid that makes your muscles sore, so if you prevent this chemical reaction from taking place, you can prevent sore muscles. In this case, more is not better. Rest between sets.

Even with exercise, it is important to know when to stop. If you are doing your exercises, with or without your therapist, and your muscles start to burn, it is time to stop. Rest a few seconds and then resume. Just because it says, "Do ten times" on your home exercise sheet, do not push yourself to ten if your muscles start to burn or quiver. Build up to doing ten at a time. The same is true when you start your second or third set of ten. If you can only get up to six on the second set, fine. Stop. Try to get to seven the next time you do the exercises. Slow, steady progress prevents your muscles from getting too sore, while still building up your strength.

Again, the most important thing to do to keep muscle atrophy (weakening) and blood clots from occurring is to keep moving, through walking and exercise. You need to look at your total hip replacement rehabilitation as your full time job for the first six weeks at least. It is your job to get up and walk around. It is your job to do your exercises. It is not a frivolous request. It is essential in the complete rehabilitation of your hip. If you did not desire a second chance at a more functional and pain-free life, you would not have chosen to undergo the surgery in the first place. But the surgery is just the first step, probably the easiest for you because you are really not involved. Your work starts after the surgery is complete, and the more you put into it, the more you'll get out of it.

While your exercise program may look too simple and basic to really be doing anything, remember that it is accomplishing much. The basic exercises, in sitting, standing, and lying down, all help to rebuild your muscles in ways that do not put any additional stresses on your new hip. Simplicity is not a bad thing. Rest assured that if you do your exercises on a daily basis as directed by your therapist, your recovery will be smoother, quicker, and have fewer complications than if you neglect these exercises.

Chapter 15

Home Care

Getting back home adds a whole new set of complications. Hospitals and rehabilitation centers are set up to take care of people with medical problems. At home you may need to do the planning and supervision of your helpers by yourself. You will probably be working with a home care nurse, a physical therapist, and, perhaps, a home health aide. Here are some thoughts on returning home successfully.

You will probably have a home care nurse for at least part of your recovery. The nurse is an expert in the medical aspects of total hip replacement. Be honest about how you are feeling when she asks so that she will be able to assess your condition accurately. She can't help you if she doesn't know there is a problem. Be sure to ask her all of the questions that you have. Your nurse can also contact your surgeon for you if you are having trouble getting an answer or response from his office.

The physical therapist will be responsible for making sure that you continue your program of exercise after you get home. As stated earlier in this book, you cannot speed the healing of the muscles and joint capsule around your hip, but you can strengthen them. Exercise is now the predominant factor in physical therapy, but any difficulties that you are having with mobility will also be addressed.

Getting in and out of bed, not only because of muscle weakness, but also from the total hip replacement precautions, can be something that takes quite a while to master. Even when you are getting around nicely with your walker or cane, you may still need assistance getting in and out of bed. This is totally normal and to be expected. The muscles that pull your leg out to the side to get your leg off the bed, the abductor muscles, are the very muscles that the surgeon needed to cut through to get to your hip. These muscles, therefore, take the greatest time to heal and strengthen.

Another difficult task is getting in and out of the shower. If an occupational therapist does not go over this with you, the physical therapist will. Hopefully you have already taken care of the shower and the bathroom as discussed in Chapter 8. The therapist will just be making sure that you know how to use the shower after you understand the reality of your limitations.

The home health aides are there to assist with the things you cannot do at the moment. They can help you with grooming, personal hygiene, sponge baths, or assisting in getting you in and out of the shower once you have been taught by your therapist. They can also assist you with getting dressed, especially your pants, socks, and shoes which you cannot do yourself. They can clean up the area in which you are residing by vacuuming, changing the sheets, and putting out the trash. Other jobs they can do including making your breakfast or lunch, doing the dishes, and washing your clothes. The duties aides are allowed to perform vary depending on the agency and state laws, so the discharge planner at the hospital or the nurse will let you know just what the aide can do for you.

Make sure that if your insurance company is paying for an aide for two hours, you get those two hours. If the aide is late, make sure she makes up the time. Two hours can go very quickly. It takes at least that long to do a load of laundry from start to finish. You are entitled to get what you pay for, so contact the agency with any time discrepancies or problems. Have a list of things you need done available and, if the aide is sitting in front of the TV because she says she's done everything already, start reading from the list. Use the aide while she's there. That is what she is being paid for, not sitting and watching "The View."

Chapter 16

Outpatient Physical Therapy

Once you are capable of getting in and out of the car without much difficulty, you will be ready for outpatient physical therapy. Treatments usually last about an hour and require that you get to and from the office two to three times per week for treatments. It really doesn't matter how soon you get there. The course of treatment is the same during the first six weeks whether you are in a rehabilitation center, at home, or in outpatient therapy. There is no rushing Mother Nature and, until the six-week point when your muscles and joint capsule have had a chance to heal, therapy will be mild.

Following the initial six weeks, you can start to increase your strengthening activities. As guided by your surgeon and physical therapist, more muscle building exercises will be added to your program, including light weights and some basic exercise machines. During your entire rehabilitation, do not forget about working your arms. You can use weights right from the start if you are up to it. Slow progression is the key with all rehabilitation. Remember that your body will let you overdo, but that you will pay for it the next day.

Treadmills and weight machines will be added to your program as seen fit by your therapist. Biking, because it forces your hip past 90 degrees of flexion, may be withheld for a few more weeks. When you start on the stationary bike, the seat will be up as high as possible to decrease the flexion at your hip when pedaling. Time on the bike and treadmill will be low in the beginning, but try to increase your time on each visit. Remember that you probably were not very active before surgery or during the first six weeks post-op. Set small personal goals and celebrate when you achieve each one.

If pain or swelling is a problem, your therapist can address these issues. Make sure you maintain an open line of communication with your therapist. More than likely, you will work with both a physical therapist and a physical therapy assistant. Make sure you feel comfortable with the therapist or assistant with whom you are working. If there is a problem, do not hesitate to speak to someone in charge and ask for a change.

At some facilities, you may see different physical therapists throughout your rehabilitation depending on your appointment schedule. Flexibility on your part with appointments may aid you in seeing the same physical therapist or physical therapy assistant on each visit. Speak with the director of the facility if you are encountering too many new faces each week. Working with the same physical therapist or physical therapy assistant on a continuing basis helps to assure steadier progress with your program.

Honesty is always the best policy and, with rehabilitation, this is particularly true. All too often when asked how they are, people automatically say, "I'm fine, thanks" without giving much thought as to how they really feel. Make sure you tell your therapist exactly how you are feeling. Do not sugar coat anything. They know what warning signs to look for if any arise, so make sure you keep them well informed on all aspects of your rehabilitation. Working together as a team, you and your therapist will devise the best plan available to help you achieve your post-surgical goals. Follow this plan and your rehabilitation will succeed. Your responsibility is to follow through with the instructions given to you by your therapist. Working out on machines two to three times a week is not enough. You need to continue with your daily exercise program when you are not at therapy and use your therapy sessions as an adjunct to this program.

Although many people incorporate outpatient physical therapy into their rehabilitation plan, sometimes people do not feel the need to continue with outpatient therapy following the therapy they received in the rehabilitation center or home care. Depending on your insurance coverage and how you are doing post-operatively, you might only be eligible for a week or two of home care. Sometimes additional therapy is needed. Other times, it is not. Each person is different. What works for some does not work for all. The decision to continue with therapy on an outpatient basis must be made based on the needs of the individual. For example, someone who is older and has led a sedentary lifestyle for many years and does not plan on doing any strenuous or sport activities with the new hip may not feel the need to continue on with outpatient therapy following the termination of home care. Continuing with a home exercise program on a daily basis might be all that is required to maintain the strength and flexibility needed. On the other hand, someone who is planning to return to a more active lifestyle, including participating in sports, may want to take the extra time to finish rehabilitation, including progressing to a more strenuous exercise program, in outpatient physical therapy.

Chapter 17

Helpful Hints

Through the years, I have discovered many helpful hints that I share with my patients. They range from how to get out of bed more easily to the best way of getting into a car. My philosophy is the more information you are armed with, the better off you are, and the more successful your rehabilitation.

Getting in and out of Bed

Getting in bed and getting out of bed can be two of the most difficult challenges you face following total hip replacement surgery. It is easier to get in and out of bed on the opposite side of your operated leg. For example, if you had your right hip replaced, then you would want to enter and exit the bed on the left side (left as if you were facing the headboard). This allows your unoperated leg to get up onto the bed first so you can use it to help raise your operated leg. This can be done by lying on your back,

bending the knee of the unoperated leg, and pressing the
foot down into the bed while lifting the operated leg. More
than likely, you will need assistance with this for some
time. The person assisting you can gently raise your leg up
to the bed level by holding your ankle and behind your
knee as shown in Figure 15. Make sure your assistants use
proper body mechanics and lift with their legs and not their
back. The last thing you need is for your assistants to be out
of commission with a back injury. See Figure 16 for an
example of how NOT to lift a leg.

Getting out of bed is also tricky. The movement of
bringing your leg away from your body (abduction) is
difficult because the surgeon cut through this muscle group.

You may need help getting out of bed for a few weeks.
The person who assists you will generally hold your leg at
the ankle and slowly and gently glide your leg to the side of

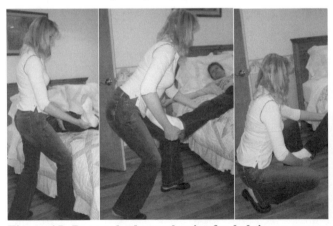

**Figure 15: Proper body mechanics for helping a person
get out of bed. Keep the back straight and use your legs.**

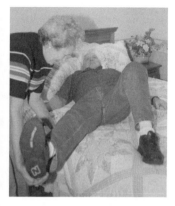

Figure 16: If you are the helper, don't bend at the back when you are lifting a leg. You might end up with a back injury. Bend your legs to do the lifting.

the bed for or with you. Figure 15 shows how to do this with good body mechanics.

As your muscles get stronger, ask your assistant to do less, while you progressively do more. Eventually, you will be able to get in and out of bed on your own, but do not let it get you down if this takes a while. It is totally normal and expected.

Climbing the Stairs

Going up is harder physically, but coming down is more difficult psychologically. Whenever you use the stairs right after surgery, you will want to have someone with you for safety. That person should always stay on the downhill side of you. For example, when you are going up the stairs, your assistant is behind you. Coming down the stairs, your assistant is in front of you. This is done so that if you lose your balance downward, your assistant just gives you a little push and the worst that happens is that you sit on a step (versus tumbling down the stairs).

In the health care field, we never like to use the terms "bad" leg or "good" leg for your operated and non-operated legs respectively. However, for this next helpful hint, we are going to break that rule. Whenever you are doing the stairs, use this mnemonic to help you remember which foot goes first: Up with the good — good people go up to Heaven, and down with the bad — bad people go down to

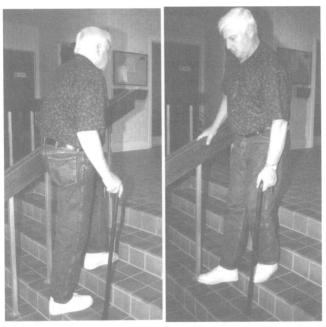

Figure 17: Going up the stairs with the "good" leg first. Coming down with the "bad" leg first.

you-know-where! (See Figure 17.) With this little phrase running through your head, you will have no problem remembering which leg goes first.

Even without the phrase, it will be plain to see which leg goes up the stairs first. If you attempt to put your operated foot up on the step first while going up the stairs, you will feel some strain and, more than likely, your operated leg will be too weak to lift your entire body up onto the next step.

Don't try to force anything. Just put your operated leg back down and put the non-operated leg up to make the climb. Likewise, when you are going down the stairs, if you leave your operated leg to go down last, it will have to lower your entire body weight onto the next step and you will feel it. It is not likely you will make these mistakes often. Your body has a way of telling you how to do things the right way and letting you know when you have screwed up.

Getting in and out of the Car

Following a total hip replacement, getting in and out of a car can be tough, especially while maintaining the total hip replacement precautions. The best seat to ride in is the passenger seat, pushed back as far as possible. You will also need to put a pillow or other type of cushion on the seat to raise the level of the seat. Then take this pillow with you to also elevate whatever seat you sit in once you get to your destination. (Most orthopedic offices have at least one elevated chair now, but you would be surprised how many office waiting rooms do not even have one seat appropriate for their own patients.)

To get into the car, open the door and back into the seat area with your walker or other assistive device. Then reach back with both hands for something solid and stable. This can be the dashboard, back of the seat, car frame, anything except the door. The door can move, so it is best to avoid touching the door at all, much less grabbing it for support. Once you have your hands in place, straighten out your operated leg and place it forward ahead of your body and then lower your bottom onto the seat. Slide back on the seat towards the driver's side. You may use your non-operated leg on the car door frame to help push yourself back.

Next lean backwards towards the driver's side while slowly and gently bringing your legs, one at a time into the car. By leaning back, you decrease the degree of bend at your waist, giving you the room to lift your leg up to get it into the car and over the door frame without bending at the waist part 90 degrees. When bringing your leg into the car, think of a frog to keep your leg from rotating inward. If your operated leg is your left leg, your knee must enter the car before your foot. If your operated leg is the right leg, your foot must enter first. Picture a frog's legs in your head. Can you see it? Once your legs are in the car, you can then straighten up and belt yourself in because you are ready to roll.

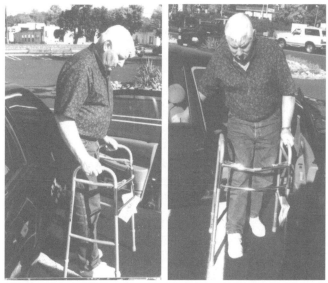

Figure 18: Positioning the walker and finding a solid place to hold on.

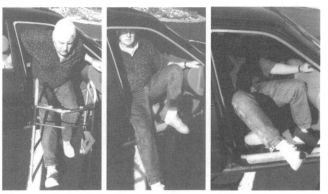

Figure 19: Lowering yourself into the car and pushing back into the seat with the "frog leg" technique.

Getting out of the car is much like getting in, only in reverse. You still want to think of a frog when bringing your legs out of the car. First lean back towards the driver's side. Then slowly bring out your right leg. If this is your operated leg, you will need to bring your knee out before your foot. Then comes the left leg. If this is your operated leg, your foot comes first, followed by your knee. When both legs are out of the car, slide forward on the seat, extend your operated leg so that your knee is straight and lower than your hip, grab onto any part of the car that does not move, and lean slightly forward to get up. Have the driver place your walker or assistive device in front of you and then you are off. Piece of cake!

If you have trouble with the pivoting and sliding part of getting into a car, try putting a large plastic garbage bag on the seat to help you slide more easily. You may also need assistance getting your operated leg into and out of the car. As time goes on, this will become easier and you will eventually be able to do more and more by yourself.

As you can probably tell from this description, you are not just jumping into your car and zooming off. It takes a few minutes to transfer into the car and then get your assistive device tucked away before you drive off. Make sure you allow extra time for this, especially when you are going to a doctor's appointment. More mistakes happen when people rush than any other time. Factor in the extra time and you will all be happier for the effort.

Hurting Heels

If you find that your heels are getting sore from lying on your back, place a small, rolled-up towel under your ankles to lift your heels slightly off the mattress. Make sure that your feet continue to comply with the total hip replacement precautions and roll outward. You can also do ankle pumps in bed by pointing your toes and then bringing them up again as if waving with your feet. (No side to side movement!) This will help with blood flow. Tell your doctor about any areas of redness on your heels that do not go away within 15 minutes of getting up out of bed.

Your Attitude

The rehabilitation from your total hip replacement can be either agony or a satisfying challenge depending almost entirely upon your attitude. If you constantly want everything to be done yesterday, you are in for a long six weeks. However, if you look at each stage of your rehabilitation as a new and conquerable challenge, your rehabilitation will be much smoother and more successful.

Over the years of my practice, I have found that patients who set several small goals for themselves rather than grandiose ones have a more tolerable rehabilitation period. When you set smaller goals, doable in less time, you have a greater sense of accomplishment. I encourage my patients to set small goals with short time frames. Then when you accomplish that goal, celebrate it. This approach lends itself to a greater feeling of accomplishment and pride. You will be eager to progress to the next goal. Your determination and dedication is strengthened and your rehabilitation reaps the rewards.

Larger goals that require more time to complete can be discouraging. You may not see small progress, but only look at what you still can't do. Focusing on the negative does nothing to motivate you. Less exercise and walking are done because you do not feel it is doing anything for you. I often tell my patients that they are not able to see progress well on a day-to-day basis because they are living with themselves and cannot see it. I encourage them to look at their progress on more of a week-to-week basis. Usually the differences from one week to the next are so visible, even the most critical skeptics have to admit advancement.

Handling Depression

Depression following major surgery is not that uncommon. If you find yourself in a negative state of mind that you cannot shake, including feelings of hopelessness, changes in eating habits, difficulty sleeping, no motivation to do your prescribed exercises or walking, call your physician immediately. Medication to help control depression can help significantly with your rehabilitation. Depression is a medical condition, just like pneumonia, and it should be treated as such. It is not a sign of weakness or failure. Treatment is available and depression is curable. Do not be afraid or ashamed to call for help if this situation arises. That call can make all the difference in the world.

Chapter 18

The Rest of Your Life

Many people worry that by having a hip replacement, their lives will be limited forever. The truth is that without the surgery, limitation is inevitable and increasing. The first few months following surgery are restricted, but the remainder of your life does not need to be. Once the joint capsule has healed and your muscles have strengthened, your hip will be better than it has been in a long time. Activities abandoned years ago because of pain are now possible once again. If you don't believe this yet, it may be time to go back and read the stories in Chapter 2 again.

Common sense is a must when you start to get back to things you used to enjoy prior to your hip problems. Some adjustments may need to be made when trying new things, especially during the first six months to a year. Research indicates that if you are able to avoid dislocating your hip for 12 months, your chances of dislocation after that are about the same as if you never had a hip replacement. The key is listening to your body and not trying to do too much.

It is normal to have some ongoing pain after the operation. The most troubling is pain related to the scar. It will be noticeable for four months or so. The problem is that it can be hard to tell whether the pain you are experiencing is from the scar or the hip joint because the scar goes all the way down to the joint itself. If it is more than a mild ache, call your doctor.

You will probably also experience some mild aches or pains in two other places off and on during the first six months. The first is somewhere near the middle of the thigh. This is normal as the bone and nerves heal. The second is near the top of the hip bone (iliac crest). You haven't used the muscles that attach here for a long time and they are going to be stiff and sore when you start using them again. Again a mild ache is probably nothing to worry about. But if you have any kind of sharp pain or a pain that lasts more than a day, discuss it with your doctor.

In general, you will be able to work yourself back into shape for almost any activity. Take your time though, to build up your strength and endurance. Although your hip is new, the rest of your body is more than likely the original model, so you need to keep that in mind.

Different people will have different activities that interest them, but one activity that many people ask about is resuming sexual relations. Your doctor will be able to tell you what is best for you, but sometimes it can be embarrassing to ask. Here are the general rules so you will be better prepared when you talk to him. A good time to ask is at your six-week follow-up exam.

You should refrain from sexual intercourse for six to eight weeks following total hip replacement surgery. Hip dislocation is a concern right after surgery, but after your surgery has healed completely, intercourse is safe. In fact, many people enjoy the experience more following recovery from their surgery because they no longer have hip discomfort or stiffness.

Most patients, male and female, prefer to resume sexual intercourse from the bottom position. This is the preferred position because you can be more careful about where you place your hips and it takes less energy.

The major concern is to find positions that follow the total hip precautions. Avoid too much bending and rotation of the hips. AboutJoints.com says the standard position is usually okay, as long as the hip is in a safe position. If the man is on the bottom, he should keep his knees slightly apart. Good communication will help make the experience safe. For more information you might want to look at http://www.aboutjoints.com/patientinfo/topics/ sexualconcerns/approvedpositions.htm

Other people are more concerned about outdoor sports. Usually you can work up to your favorite sport very soon after the six-week recovery is over. However, some sports, depending on your knowledge and skill level prior to surgery, may remain off limits for a year or more. For example, if you skied and want to return to the slopes, a slow start might be called for. It would not, however, be a good time to try to learn how to ski. Some surgeons forbid sports like skiing and golf, but depending on your age and prior skill level, a slow and slightly modified return may be possible. Tennis is another active sport that requires much twisting and bending. Although you will make it back to the courts in a few months, many surgeons recommend playing doubles instead of singles and starting off very light. Be sure to check with your surgeon before starting any sports activities.

The most common long-term complication following a total hip replacement is the loosening of the joint. Surgical techniques have improved greatly over the past two decades, adding a longer life expectancy to the integrity of the joint, but there are always the exceptions. Too many forceful stresses on the joint itself may hasten any loosening. Caution should always linger in the minds of hip replacement recipients, not to prevent movement, but more to guide and monitor what is done.

Once your new hip is healed and your hip musculature strengthened, you will be able to live a more active, less pain-filled life. This surgery has improved countless lives over the years and will continue to do so in the years to come.

Simple things that most people take for granted, like walking in the park or picking up a grandchild, are often only a distant memory for many arthritis sufferers. Following this surgery, things once taken for granted and then impossible to do, become not only possible, but also a joy. What was lost has now been found and there is really no better feeling in the world. Just remember to take is slow, as your body will let you overdo and you will pay for it.

Chapter 19

The Caregiver

Although this book is primarily for the individual who will be having the surgery, anyone who will be caring for that individual has about as much invested in the surgery as the hip replacement recipient. Reading this book will help to give you a better understanding of what to expect both for yourself and your loved one.

First off, you will be not only an emotional support; you will also be a physical assistant. Your job will start by understanding the demands and responsibilities that will fall upon your shoulders in the weeks to come. It is not an overwhelming task if you work with your partner to ensure the surgery and rehabilitation are successful.

The first way in which you can help your partner is in the decision-making process. The reality of surgery can be very frightening and intimidating. You may need to lend your moral support for this life-changing decision to be made. Encouragement and empathy are a plus and in some cases a must. Reassuring your partner that you will be with him or her through the entire process will go a long way toward helping with the final decision.

You can also help with preparations before surgery, as described in the checklists. Here are some of the most important things for you to do. Have stair railings and safety bars installed if needed. Arrange a visit to the local rehabilitation centers before surgery to assist your partner with post-hospital decisions. Clean the home and make sure that no clutter accumulates, especially on the stairs. Make sure that a hospital bed has been ordered if a bedroom is on the second floor and stairs are problematic. Install a hand-held showerhead for easy bathing and consider taking down any glass doors on tubs and replacing them with shower curtains temporarily. Review the chapter on safety and implement whatever you can to ensure a safe rehabilitation environment at home. In many small ways, what you do before surgery can make a big difference afterwards.

At the hospital and rehabilitation center, you can function as your partner's advocate if your partner is unwilling or unable to speak up on his or her own. Many people fear making waves, even when their own health and well being are on the line. If you see that something is not right, speak up immediately. You know your partner better than any of the personnel at the hospital, including the doctors, so do not hesitate to act if you think there is a problem. If you are not satisfied with the results, continue up the ladder until you get an answer or solution you can live with. Call on the hospital's patient advocate to help you solve problems quickly.

When your partner gets home, you will have several responsibilities on a physical level. Your partner will have difficulty for some time getting in and out of bed due to the area of the incision and the muscles that have been weakened by the surgery. Assisting your partner by lifting and lowering the operated leg will be one of your biggest jobs. The mere act of getting in and out of bed is no longer simple after a total hip replacement and you may find yourself assisting with this task longer than anything else. Remember to help only as much as is needed. Let the hip replacement recipient do as much as possible and fill in where necessary. You can put your hands under the heel and behind the knee of the operated leg when lifting or lowering the leg. Be careful to keep the toes pointing upward or out to the side to prevent the leg from rotating inward. Make sure to watch your own body mechanics. The last thing your partner needs is for you to be out of commission with a back injury. Use your legs, not your back, when lifting. Try not to twist your body. Move your feet rather than twisting at the waist.

If you are worried about doing something wrong, don't be. Your partner will let you know if something does not feel right. Be gentle and follow the precautions listed in this book and all will be fine.

It is hard to remember all that is thrown at you after a surgery like this, so it will be up to you to give gentle reminders to your partner when necessary. If your partner is not getting up enough, do not bring water the next time your partner asks for it. Suggest that he or she get up and get it for himself or herself. There are ways to get around nagging if you think creatively. Remember that doing too much for your partner is not helping, but may actually hinder rehabilitation. As time goes on, try to do less yourself and allow your partner to do more on his or her own. Of course, common sense must be used when enforcing this. If it is nighttime and your partner is particularly tired, it would be wise to go and get the water yourself.

Make sure that your partner gets dressed every day. Staying in nightclothes makes people feel like they are sick. The simple act of being dressed does so much for the mental well being of the hip replacement recipient. You will need to help with socks and shoes for at least the first six weeks. Assistive devices are available to help get socks on, but they are not easy to use. Elastic laces are also helpful, allowing your partner to slip into his or her shoes without having to untie and then tie the laces. These laces can be purchased at any medical supply store or online, if they have not been provided in the hospital or rehabilitation setting. A long-handled shoehorn also goes a long way in helping your partner get his or her shoes on independently.

Frustration is an issue that you will probably have to deal with at one point or another, either yours, your partners, or the both of you. The long wait for the end of the precaution stage can sometimes be very frustrating for the hip replacement recipient. Your partner is starting to feel better than he or she has in years. It's very natural to want to do more, but it doesn't mean your partner should or can. You need to remind your partner about the limitations without sounding like a know-it-all. Try to emphasize the positive. For example, remind your partner that there are only two more weeks until the next doctor's appointment and some of the restrictions will probably be lifted then. Don't be surprised if some of the frustrations get taken out on you. You are there, after all, and are the likely target of a little venting. Knowing this in advance may help you to deal with it if it occurs. Like you tell your partner, only a few more weeks and then things will surely be looking up.

If your partner is frustrated by a lack of progress, have him or her look back a week or more and compare what it was like then with the present. Sometimes, it is not possible to see advancement on a day-to-day basis because you are too close to the situation. You need to look at a wider time frame to see how far you have actually come. Help your partner to set small, attainable goals in rehabilitation and celebrate each time one of the milestones is achieved. Multiple, small goals are more beneficial than one big ultimate goal that takes weeks or months to achieve.

To ease your frustration, make sure to take advantage of all the services provided to you by the home care agency and community. If a home health aide has been assigned, use that time as your time to relax and escape the role of caretaker. It is important for both of you that you maintain your own emotional and physical well being while caring for all of your partner's needs. Meals On Wheels and other such programs may be available to you. Some ambulance squads loan equipment free of charge. Check with your nurse or the public health nurse for your town to find out more about what is available.

Be sure to watch for any signs of depression. Lack of motivation, lethargy, feelings of hopelessness, sleeping problems, and changes in appetite are some of the key symptoms of this condition. If you notice any of these symptoms in your partner that last longer than a day or so, call your doctor or nurse. Depression is a very real condition that can be successfully treated with medication. If left unchecked, depression can lead to serious consequences during rehabilitation, including muscle atrophy and blood clots.

Make sure that the therapist, either in the rehabilitation center or at home, instructs you on how to properly assist with transfers, such as getting your partner in and out of the shower and car. Even when your partner feels ready to take a shower alone, try to stay nearby for safety. Remember that most falls occur in the bathroom. If you have any questions about where to stand or what to do, make sure you ask the therapist to review it with you again.

Although you are not the one who just underwent major surgery, your job in the rehabilitation of your partner is a very important one. The benefits that your partner will reap as a result of this surgery will be more than enough of a reward for all of your efforts.

Chapter 20

Sample Exercise Programs

The following exercise programs are the basic building blocks to your rehabilitation, but don't wait until your rehabilitation to start doing them. They are simple, uncomplicated exercises in three positions: sitting, standing, and lying down. They are specifically aimed at enhancing and strengthening the muscles of you hip and leg.

Of course, this is like any other exercise program. You need to check with your doctor before you start to be sure that these exercises are appropriate for your condition.

Performing these exercises prior to surgery does two things: First, it familiarizes you with the exercises so you are not trying them for the first time immediately after surgery and, second, by doing these exercises prior to surgery, you are strengthening your hip and leg muscles, which will assist in your rehabilitation following the surgery. The stronger your legs and hip muscles are before the surgery, the easier and quicker your rehabilitation will be.

As with all exercise, you should start slow. Even if these exercise programs seem too easy, it is best to start with only one or two sets of ten repetitions and build your way up to three sets. Whenever you add weights into the equation, either for the first time or by adding more weight, it is best to return to one set of ten and then gradually build yourself up to three sets of ten. When three sets of ten become too easy, it is time to add weight. As was explained in the chapter on the importance of exercise, your body will let you overdo, so although something might appear easy, follow the rules above to ensure your best workout without soreness.

Remember to gear changes in your exercise program to what you did one day and how you feel the following morning. Again, if you awake with no or limited muscle soreness, then you can increase your activity a bit. If you wake up with some muscle soreness, but nothing over-whelming, then you probably should stay at the current level for the time being. If you awake with great discom-fort, then you have probably done too much and you should reduce your activity level, including your exercise program, by a small degree and see how you feel the next day. This day-to-day process ensures that you are progressing on a level that is right for you on an individual basis.

As mentioned earlier, do not continue with any exer-cise if you feel pain. Pain is an indicator and you must listen to your body. If you experience pain with any of the exercises, stop. Please remember that pain is subjective and therefore means different things to different people. What may be excruciating to one person may be barely annoying to another. For the purpose of exercise and pain, you need to recognize the difference between muscle soreness and pain that signals tissue damage. In general, pain is sudden, sharp and comes and goes quickly. Muscle soreness tends to be less severe, more of an achiness, and it lasts longer. Everyone is different, so you must determine the difference for yourself and base your responses accordingly.

Sometimes a muscle has a spasm during exercise. If this is the case, stop immediately and let the spasm pass. It does not do your muscles any good to exercise through a spasm. If you do the exercise again later and you still have pain, do not continue until you have consulted with your surgeon or a physical therapist.

Remember to breathe while you exercise. Now, you might think that this is silly — everyone has to breathe, right? Just for a moment, imagine that you are opening a jar and the lid is stuck. What is the first thing you do? Take a deep breath, hold it, and try to pop the top. It is a natural response to hold your breath when doing something strenuous. That is why it is a good idea to count aloud or hum while exercising. If you are speaking or humming, you must be breathing!

When you hold your breath, the pressure within your chest rises, collapsing the large vein that is bringing blood back to your heart from your organs and the lower half of your body. The problem arises when you release your breath and the sudden surge of blood that had been prevented from getting to the heart due to the collapsed vessel rushes to the heart and puts added stress on the heart to pump faster and harder. This is when a heart attack can occur. It is best to breathe normally while exercising or doing anything strenuous to ensure that this phenomenon, called a Valsalva maneuver, does not happen.

Listed below are the sample exercise programs. These programs focus primarily on your legs, but feel free to incorporate arm exercises into your workout if your doctor thinks that is appropriate. If you have any problems understanding what to do or are confused in any way about these exercises, please ask a physical therapist to assist you. You are not expected to know these exercises prior to surgery and you will be instructed in exercises just like these by your physical therapist in the hospital or home setting. Knowing these prior to surgery just puts you a little ahead of the game.

Sitting Exercises

(Best done while sitting in an elevated chair with an armrest)

1. Tap your feet as if to music. Do 10 to 30 seconds many times a day. This helps to prevent blood clots in your legs.

2. Slowly straighten out your knee and then bend it again. Do 10 times.

3. Put your hands on the armrest of your chair and slowly lift your bottom up off the chair slightly. Then lower yourself again. Do 5 times. (This exercise helps strengthen the muscles you need to get up out of a chair)

4. Bring you hands up to chest level and slowly punch out in front of you, alternating arms. Do 10 times.

5. Put your arms out to the side. Keeping your arms straight, slowly raise your arms up over your head and then lower them again slowly. Do 10 times.

Remember to breathe. Stop if you have any pain!

Bed Exercises

(Best done lying flat on your back or slightly propped up on pillows)

1. Bend your knee, keeping your foot flat on the bed, and slide your heel up towards your bottom. Then slowly lower your leg again. Do 10 times. (Do not go past 90 degrees at your hip)

2. Bring your leg out to the side and back in again slowly. Do not cross the midline of your body. Do 10 times. (You may find it easier, especially after surgery, to bend your unoperated leg, keeping that foot flat on the bed, while trying to move the operated leg out to the side.)

3. Bend both knees, placing your feet flat on the bed. Slowly lift your bottom slightly off the bed and hold for a slow count of five while breathing in and out. Then lower yourself slowly. Do 10 times.

4. Bend up one knee, placing the foot flat on bed, and keep the other leg straight. Slowly lift and lower the straight leg up off the bed 6" to 8". Do 10 times.

5. Wave your feet back and forth at your ankle joint. Do 10 to 30 seconds many times a day. (Be sure not to let your foot turn inward)

Standing Exercises

(Best done by standing and holding onto something sturdy and permanent, like the kitchen sink)

1. Bring your leg out to the side and back in again. Do 10 times. (Make sure that you are standing up tall and bringing your leg straight out to the side. You should feel the muscle working in your hip and buttocks area.)

2. Bring your leg back behind you and back in again. Do 10 times. (This is not a big movement. Make sure that you do not lean forward, but rather remain standing up straight.)

3. Raise yourself up onto your toes and then lower yourself slowly. Do 10 times. Do not rock back onto your heels.

4. March in place by lifting one leg up at a time. Do 10 times. (Do not pass 90 degrees while marching. Keep your knee lower than your hip.)

5. Bend your knees slightly and then straighten up again. Do 10 times. (Make sure that you stick out your buttocks as if you were going to sit in a chair when bending your knees. When you look down, your knees should not pass in front of your toes.)

Glossary of Terms

abduction: The movement of a body part away from the midline of the body.

abduction pillow: A triangular pillow used to keep the legs separated following total hip replacement surgery. This pillow frequently has eight long straps coming from it that attach around the patient's legs to keep the pillow in place.

acetabulum: The part of the iliac or pelvis bone that forms the cup or socket into which the femoral head fits, forming the hip joint.

adduction: The movement of a body part toward the midline of the body.

atrophy: The weakening of muscles from lack of use.

avascular necrosis: A condition in which the blood flow to the head of the femur is diminished, causing the bone cells to die. The bone becomes weakened and very often fractures or breaks.

extension: The straightening of a limb at the joint.

femur: The large bone in the thigh that runs between the hip and knee.

femoral head: The round, ball-shaped end of the femur that comes together with the acetabulum (socket) to form the hip joint, a ball and socket joint.

femoral neck: The long, thin section of the femur that runs between the femoral head and the thick main shaft of the bone. Because of its design, this is a common site of hip fractures.

flexion: The act of bending at a joint.

full weight bearing: A term used to indicate that one's full body weight is allowed on the operated leg.

general anesthesia: The administration of medications that render the body completely unconscious so that surgery can be performed. Patients under general anesthesia lose the ability to move, feel, and even breathe on their own. Breathing is assisted with a ventilator.

ileum: The bone that makes up the greatest portion of your pelvis. The acetabulum (socket of the hip joint) is a part of this bone.

joint: The connection where two or more bones come together.

ligament: Fibrous tissue that connects bone to bone.

regional anesthesia: The administration of drugs directly to the nervous system to eliminate pain, feeling, and movement from a specific area of the body. When used during surgery, the patient can remain awake during the procedure.

nosocomial infection: An infection that occurs as a result of being in a hospital. The germs are in the hospital and are passed along to you during your stay.

non-weight bearing: A term used to indicate that no weight at all is allowed on the operated leg or specific limb.

orthopedic surgeon: A surgeon who specializes in operating on bones and joints. Further specialization exists within this group, sub-specialties such as hand surgeon, knee surgeon, etc.

partial weight bearing: A term used to indicate less than full weight bearing, usually a percentage of total body weight. For example, 20% weight bearing for a person weighing 150 pounds would be only 30 pounds of pressure allowed on that limb while walking.

rehabilitation center: An inpatient center that specializes in rehabilitation.

tendon: The thin ends of a muscle, which attach it to bone.

toe-touch weight bearing: A confusing term that indicates minimal weight bearing allowed on the operated leg or involved limb.

Index

Master Checklist Before Surgery

☐	I read the stories of other people who have had total hip replacement surgery and I want to consider this option. (Chapter 2)
☐	I found a doctor for my surgery whom I like and trust. (Chapter 3)
☐	I selected the hospital where I will have my surgery. (Chapter 4)
☐	I have given my doctor all of the information he needs to make sure my surgery will be successful. (Chapter 5)
☐	I have scheduled my surgery. (Chapter 5)
☐	I understand how much my insurance will cover and am ready to pay for the rest. (Chapter 6)
☐	I have picked my rehabilitation center after surgery. OR
☐	I plan to go home right after the hospital. (Chapter 7)
☐	I have found home health care workers to take care of me after I get home. (Chapter 7)
☐	I selected a facility for outpatient physical therapy. OR
☐	I'm going to wait to see how I feel after surgery before I decide on outpatient physical therapy. (Chapter 7)

More

Master Checklist Before Surgery (continued)

☐	My home is ready for me, so I will be comfortable there after my surgery. (Chapter 8)
☐	I understand the total hip precautions and I will follow them carefully after my surgery. (Chapter 9)
☐	I understand the surgery procedure as well as I want to. (Chapter 10)
☐	I understand what will happen after surgery. (Chapters 11 to 18)

Master Checklist for Your Hospital Stay

☐	I know who my nurse is for each shift.
☐	I am insisting on good care, while still respecting my caregivers.
☐	I am taking my pain medication. It's keeping the pain under control. It's not too strong or making me feel funny.
☐	I survived the first day after surgery.
☐	And I got on my feet!
☐	I know how much weight I can put on my new hip. My limit is _____.
☐	I can use a walker or crutches.
☐	I can get in and out of a chair.
☐	When someone helps, I can get in and out of bed.
☐	(If you had general anesthesia) The effects of the anesthesia are wearing off and I am thinking as well as before the surgery.
☐	I understand the total hip replacement precautions and I plan to follow them.
☐	My therapists and doctors have told me all the information I need to have a safe and healthy recovery. And I understood what they told me.
☐	My physical therapist gave me some exercises.
☐	My occupational therapist showed me how to use the adaptive equipment that I need during recovery.
☐	Before leaving I gathered up all of the equipment that I am entitled to take with me.
☐	I shared my thoughts with the hospital.

Master Checklist for Recovery

☐	I know how much weight I am allowed to put on my leg.
☐	I transferred to a rehabilitation center.
☐	I am doing what the physical therapist tells me to do.
☐	I went home!
☐	The home care nurse is following the progress of my recovery.
☐	I am doing what the home care physical therapist tells me to do.
☐	My home health aide is seeing to my needs as required. Any concerns have been adequately addressed by the aide or the agency.
☐	I can get in and out of a car.
☐	I made it through my first trip back to the doctor (or outpatient rehab).
☐	I can climb stairs (and go down, too).
☐	Getting in and out of bed is getting easier.
☐	I can use a cane instead of a walker.
☐	I can get in and out of bed by myself.
☐	I can walk on my own without any assistive devices!
☐	I finished my six-week recovery successfully.
☐	Now I'm going to outpatient physical therapy to get myself in shape to do the things I really want to be able to do.
☐	I can get out and do things I haven't done in years, but I promise to be sensible about what I do.

Week by Week Checklist for Recovery

Task	1	2	3	4	5	6
I am remembering to get up and move around every hour.	☐	☐	☐	☐	☐	☐
I am tapping my feet frequently to improve blood flow to my heart.	☐	☐	☐	☐	☐	☐
I am getting out of bed and dressed every day.	☐	☐	☐	☐	☐	☐
I am getting up and walking every day.	☐	☐	☐	☐	☐	☐
I am exercising every day — not too much and never to the point of pain — but I am making progress. I can feel my strength and ability to move around coming back.	☐	☐	☐	☐	☐	☐
My attitude is good. I'm not getting too discouraged because I can set a small goal and accomplish it at least once or twice a week.	☐	☐	☐	☐	☐	☐
I understand that depression is a possibility and I know that if I get too discouraged and down, my therapist and doctor can help.	☐	☐	☐	☐	☐	☐
I am remembering to thank my caregiver at least once a week for all the help he or she is giving my throughout my recovery and rehabilitation. (Once a day might be better.)	☐	☐	☐	☐	☐	☐